APHASIOLOGY, 2003, *17* (4), 329–332

Editorial:
Quality of life in aphasia

Linda E. Worrall

The University of Queensland, Brisbane, Australia

Audrey L. Holland

The University of Arizona, USA, and The University of Queensland, Brisbane, Australia

This special issue of *Aphasiology* is dedicated to the topic of quality of life in aphasia. The issue includes a number of studies describing and measuring quality of life in people with aphasia. It also contains studies that have developed and evaluated interventions which have addressed quality of life issues in people with aphasia. Research into quality of life issues in aphasia, especially intervention studies that target quality of life in aphasia, should be a priority for clinical aphasiologists. This editorial seeks to provide a broad overview of the areas where there is consensus, and then to suggest a path forward for further research.

Quality of life measures have major implications for the development and evaluation of healthcare policies, allocation of resources, planning of future healthcare needs, implementation of health-related surveys, and evaluation of the efficacy of clinical treatments and research trials. The increase in emphasis on global health outcomes, as well as quality of life measures, results from many factors, including: (a) an increasing acknowledgment that quality of life is a crucial outcome; (b) a shift in focus from merely prolonging life to concerns with its quality; (c) growing interest and willingness to compare quality of life as affected by different medical conditions or as a result of different diseases; and (d) a general consensus about the centrality of an individuals' own perceptions of their health and life quality.

Thus in relation to aphasia as well as a host of other impairments, the study of quality of life in aphasia is burgeoning. Quality of life after aphasia is regarded as a highly significant topic for the following reasons:

• Improving quality of life is the ultimate goal of aphasia rehabilitation. Although this goal is often only implicit and addressed indirectly (e.g., improving language generalises to improved everyday communication which improves quality of life) it can also be stated explicitly and addressed directly through interventions that target the domains thought to be important for good quality of life (for example, learning to negotiate the public transportation system).

Address correspondence to: Linda E. Worrall, Associate Professor, Communication Disability in Ageing Research Unit, Department of Speech Pathology and Audiology, The University of Queensland, Brisbane, Australia. E-mail: l.worrall@uq.edu.au

© 2003 Taylor & Francis

http://www.tandf.co.uk/journals/pp/02687038.html

DOI:10.1080/02687030244000699

• Understanding clients' perspectives of their own quality of life is crucial in targeting appropriate and effective interventions. Assessing clients' quality of life therefore provides broad insights into their values, their conceptions of their own well-being and the effect that aphasia generally has had on their lives. It could therefore be considered an ideal starting point in the rehabilitation process.

• The relative impact of aphasia, compared to other impairments, can most clearly be seen through measures of quality of life. Most aphasiologists have firsthand knowledge of the devastating effect of aphasia. However, funding agencies, as well as society in general, appear to have little knowledge or appreciation of the impact of this problem. It is therefore important that the impact of aphasia on quality of life is documented and compared to other impairments.

• Measuring quality of life is a very important outcome measure that can be used for accountability purposes. Clinicians are increasingly required to show that their interventions have positive effects on everyday life for people with aphasia.

To date, speech-language pathologists have not routinely incorporated quality of life measures into standard clinical practice. However, most clinicians agree that effective communication is integral to a good quality of life. Most would also agree that enhanced quality of life is the ultimate aim of intervention, and many further believe that quality of life is compromised following the onset of aphasia. How much evidence do we have for these statements? There are other questions as well, such as the following: Is communication really as important to quality of life as we, who have chosen to work with disordered communication, might think? How can aphasia therapists place greater emphasis on quality of life issues in the management of aphasia? These are but a few examples of the issues that need to be studied in aphasiology research.

WHAT DO WE KNOW ABOUT QUALITY OF LIFE IN APHASIA?

The first conclusion from relevant research is that quality of life is negatively affected by aphasia and for the most part, this impact is significant. Nevertheless, there is no current consensus on the *extent* of the impact, particularly as aphasia might compare to other impairments. Most studies also agree that there is considerable individual variation in aphasia's impact: some affected individuals report that aphasia forms a large reason for their poorer quality of life, while for others aphasia is responsible for only a small part of their overall quality of life. Another common finding across quality of life studies in aphasia is that emotional health and well-being are important components of quality of life after aphasia. Depression, for example, is a common sequel to aphasia and must be accounted for when measuring quality of life.

Because most measures of quality of life use self-report questionnaires, it has been suggested that the language disorder itself may prevent aphasic individuals from accurately completing written questionnaires or responding validly in interviews. On that assumption many studies of quality of life in stroke or other acquired brain injuries have specifically excluded people with aphasia, or have substituted proxy evaluators instead. However, when appropriate modifications are made that enable people with aphasia to participate directly in the assessment of quality of their lives, they appear to be able to participate. Thus, techniques such as interviewing persons with aphasia rather than asking them to complete a written questionnaire unaided, simplifying questions and response formats, adding visual cues such as pictographs, using a system of prompts including personalising the question, are all helpful in enabling persons with aphasia to provide valid responses to quality of life surveys. Therefore, the second conclusion from studies in the area is that aphasic individuals, with proper attention to their communication needs, can reliably report on the quality of their lives.

WHAT DON'T WE KNOW ABOUT QUALITY OF LIFE IN APHASIA?

The use of proxies to report on quality of life issues in aphasia forms a convenient segue into what we do not know about quality of life following the onset of aphasia. In studies that use proxies, significant others are typically asked to answer the questions on behalf of the person with aphasia. There is still a lack of consensus about the validity of this approach (see Engell, Hütter, Willmes & Huber, in this issue). There is also a lack of consensus about what type of quality of life measure is most appropriate for people with aphasia. Is a subjective approach more suitable or are objective measures appropriate in some situations? Should aphasiologists be measuring health-related quality of life or psychological well-being? Are measures that emphasise motor and sensory domains inappropriate for people with aphasia because of their emphasis on physical health? An argument could be made that each different type of quality of life measurement is appropriate to the task at hand.

Although we can conclude that quality of life is important to aphasia rehabilitation, there is a lack of consensus about speech-language pathologists' roles in improving quality of life. While the American Speech-Language-Hearing Association and the Canadian Association of Speech-Language Pathologists and Audiologists Scope of Practice documents suggest that a speech-language pathologist's role is encompassed within the World Health Organisation's International Classification of Functioning, Disability and Health—ICF (2001), quality of life is not part of this conceptual framework. It lies outside the ICF, predominantly because the World Health Organisation defines quality of life as "an individual's perception of their position in life in the context of the culture and value systems in which they live and in relation to their goals, expectations, standards and concerns" (WHO, 1993, p.5), That is, for WHO purposes, quality of life remains essentially outside a focus on health. Thus, for speech-language pathologists, it is important to question how much of the reported quality of life of a person with aphasia stems from the aphasia itself, and therefore what is our role in other domains (e.g., socio-economic, physical health) that are not directly related to the aphasia? A further professional controversy is the extent of the relationship between language improvement obtained through impairment-based therapy and quality of life. Much of aphasiology is based on the premise that improvements in language have a beneficial effect on quality of life. Some preliminary research (see Cruice, Worrall, Hickson, & Murison; Hilari, Wiggins, Roy, Byng, & Smith; and Ross & Wertz, in this issue) suggests that other factors such as social relationships and participation, functional communicative ability, emotional distress, involvement in activities, and environment aspects, amongst others, may relate more strongly to quality of life. This research implies that factors other than language impairment should form the focus of intervention if improved well-being is the goal of intervention.

There are still more unknowns. Quality of life for people with severe and global aphasia is a major challenge. Creative study on how to obtain the opinions of these people is required. Methods of factoring out other variables such as depression, premorbid factors, as well as age-related concerns such as retirement, sensory and cognitive impairments, and social isolation have not been studied. Perhaps the most important issue is how to cast treatment in ways to maximise quality life post-aphasia. Examples of interventions that directly and indirectly address quality of life are required as well as high levels of evidence for their effectiveness. There are two reports of approaches in this issue (by Avent, and by Sorin-Peters) that begin to address quality of life issues. Following on from the work reported in this issue, the relative efficiency of each target of intervention also requires investigation.

CONCLUSION

In conclusion, this special issue of *Aphasiology* brings together several studies of quality of life following aphasia. Some consensus has emerged on some of the issues but there remains much research and development to be done in this most important area. It is hoped that this special issue will promote discussion and debate, and encourage researchers and clinicians alike to embrace the concept of quality of life in aphasia.

APHASIOLOGY, 2003, *17* (4), 333–353

Finding a focus for quality of life with aphasia: Social and emotional health, and psychological well-being

Madeline Cruice

University of Queensland and Royal Brisbane Hospital, Australia

Linda Worrall and Louise Hickson

University of Queensland, Australia

Robert Murison

University of Queensland, Australia

Background: Speech pathologists infrequently address the quality of aphasic people's lives in a direct manner in rehabilitation, most likely due to the difficulty in grasping the role of communication in quality of life (QOL). Despite considerable research into aphasic language impairments and communication disabilities, there is no clear evidence how aphasia impacts on clients' QOL. This paper reports on a comprehensive evaluation of 30 people with mild to moderate aphasia to determine which aspects of communication predict their QOL. A conceptual model of the relationship between communication and QOL was devised, using the disablement framework of the International Classification of Impairment, Activity and Participation Beta–2 Draft (ICIDH-2) (World Health Organisation, 1998). Communication was conceptualised as language impairment, functional communication ability and activity, and social participation. QOL included both health-related QOL (HRQOL) and psychological well-being concepts.

Aims: The aim of this study was to investigate how measures of impairment, activity and participation, and measures of QOL related to each other for people with aphasia, for the purpose of: (1) determining which specific communication assessments were most predictive of their QOL; and (2) determining whether HRQOL or psychological well-being was represented more in relationships, thus indicating a focus for QOL in aphasia.

Methods & Procedures: Thirty people aged 57–88 years (mean = 70.7yrs) with predominantly mild to moderate chronic aphasia (mean WAB AQ = 74.4, range 21.9–95.8; mean TPO = 41 mths, range 10–108 mths) participated in this study. In total, 13 standardised and specifically designed measures evaluated the different concepts of the model. Maximal multiple regression analysis illustrated which communication measures were most predictive of participants' HRQOL and psychological well-being.

Outcomes & Results: Overall, aphasic people's communication predicted their psychological well-being and social health (a subscale of HRQOL). Specifically, the findings demonstrated that functional communication ability, and language functioning to a lesser degree, were implicated in QOL, providing evidence for particular speech pathology interventions in addressing clients' QOL. Finally, emotional health powerfully influenced the relationships among variables, and physiological/physical health was a determinant of social participation.

Address correspondence to: Dr Madeline Cruice, Department of Language and Communication Science, City University, Northampton Square, London EC1V 0HB, UK. Email: m.cruice@city.ac.uk

The authors wish to thank the people with aphasia and their family members or friends who participated willingly and with interest in this study.

DOI:10.1080/0268703024400707

Conclusions: The findings suggest that aphasic people's QOL may be understood best in terms of their social participation, emotional health, and psychological well-being. Clinicians may directly target these three areas, and indirectly target them through language and functional communication, as well as targeting the contextual factors of people's lives. A new model of communication-related QOL has been devised.

It is generally assumed in life, and implicitly understood by many, that "life quality for most people is dependent upon the ability and opportunity to communicate" (Salomon, Vesterager, & Jagd, 1998, p. 164). However, a review of quality of life (QOL) literature (Cruice, Worrall, & Hickson, 2000) suggests that communication has not been investigated as a factor or determinant of QOL, most probably because of its implicitness. Consequently there is little research on how communication impairment contributes to QOL, and how the sequelae of communication disability, as well as life factors, influence people's QOL. There is a need for specific exploration into the relationship between communication and QOL, so that speech pathologists can address QOL issues in clients' communication rehabilitation with an empirically based understanding.

In speech pathology, QOL research has been undertaken primarily in five populations over the last decade: head and neck cancer populations; aphasia; Parkinson's disease; traumatic brain injury; and dysphonia (Cruice et al., 2000). Within aphasia, psychological well-being, caregiver burden, life satisfaction, and overall disability have been studied (Brumfitt, 1998; Engell, Huber, & Hütter, 1998; Hilari & Byng, 2001; Hinckley, 1998; Hoen, Thelander, & Worsley, 1997; Lyon et al., 1997; Records & Baldwin, 1996; Sarno, 1997). LaPointe (1999) provides a theoretical perspective on QOL with aphasia, based on a cancer perspective, wherein QOL is defined as a number of dimensions, some of which are less relevant for people with aphasia. Although QOL as a construct has not been researched in aphasia, the following qualitative personal studies and clinical measurement about life issues provide valuable information and insight into possible QOL with stroke and aphasia.

Stroke survivors describe the impact of their stroke on life in terms of bodily dysfunction, fatigue in activities of daily living (ADL), identity and self-esteem issues, and independence (Bendz, 2000; Buscherhof, 1998; Cant, 1997; Newborn, 1998). Findings of 12 stroke studies conclusively establish depression, physical and functional disablement, and impaired social functioning as the major issues in post-stroke QOL (Ahlsiö, Britton, Murray, & Theorelli, 1984; Aström, Asplund, & Aström, 1992; Kappelle, Adams, Hefffner, Torner, Gomez, & Biller, 1994; Kauhanen, Korpelainen, Hiltunen, Nieminen, Sotaniemi, & Myllälä, 2000; Löfgren, Gustafson, & Nyberg, 1999; Niemi, Laaksonen, Kotila, & Waltimo, 1998; Nilsson, Aniansson, & Grimby, 2000; Robinson-Smith, Johnston, & Allen, 2000; Schuling, Greidanus, & Meyboom-De Jong, 1993; Williams, Weinberger, Harris, Clark, & Biller, 1999; Wyller, Sveen, Sodring, Pettersen, & Bautz-Holter, 1997; Yoon, 1997). A recent research synthesis of 39 studies confirmed the above-mentioned three areas as dictating survivors' QOL (Bays, 2001).

People with aphasia have described the following as important to their lives: mental attitudes, emotions, sense of self, autonomy and choice, communication, relationships, social life, and community participation (Hoen et al., 1997; Le Dorze & Brassard, 1995; Zemva, 1999). Eight studies of QOL with aphasia investigated physical health, psychosocial functioning and adjustment, subjective and psychological well-being, affect, and other subjective constructs (Engell et al., 1998; Hemsley & Code, 1996; Hilari & Byng, 2001; Hinckley, 1998; Hoen et al., 1997; Lyon et al., 1996; Records & Baldwin, 1996; Sarno, 1997). Thus, collectively, physical functioning, emotional health or depression, social functioning, psychological functioning, well-being, communication, autonomy, and relationships are crucial to QOL following a stroke with aphasia. The authors arranged these dimensions of QOL into a model for this study, using the well-developed disablement framework of the World Health Organisation. This formed the basis for a concrete understanding of the relationship between communication and QOL.

The International Classification of Impairments, Activity and Participation—Revised Beta 1 and 2 Drafts (ICIDH-2) is a revised edition of the previous International Classification of Impairment, Disability and Handicap (ICIDH) from the World Health Organisation (WHO, 1998). This framework continues to be updated, and is now known as the International Classification of Functioning, Disability and Health (ICF). Beta 1 and Beta 2 Drafts were used in the conceptualisation process of this research, therefore, the *terminology* and *models* of those drafts are referred to in this paper. However, the model of the updated Beta 2 Draft is used in this paper. A brief synopsis of the ICIDH-2 is provided here.

The ICIDH-2 is a classification of "disablements", an umbrella term covering three dimensions: (1) body structures and function; (2) personal activities; and (3) participation in society (WHO, 1998). The ICIDH-2 classifies the consequences of a health condition, which is seen here as stroke with associated aphasia, in the three dimensions. In the context of a health condition (WHO, 1998, pp. 10–12):

• Impairment is a loss or abnormality of body structure or of a physiological or psychological function. Impairments are qualified by severity, localisation and duration.
• Activity is the nature and extent of functioning at the level of the person. Activities are qualified by degree of difficulty, assistance, duration and outlook.
• Participation is the nature and extent of a person's involvement in life situations in relationship to Impairments, Activities, health conditions, and contextual factors. Participation may be qualified by extent, and facilitators or barriers.

Previously based on the medical model, the ICIDH-2 combines medical, biological, and social approaches to health, and classifies the consequences associated with health conditions, in this case aphasia from stroke. Although the ICIDH-2 does not conceptualise QOL for people with health conditions, it has been used in combination with various constructs of QOL. Several models of the ICIDH–QOL relationship have been proposed and tested (Bech, 1993; Enderby, 1992; Fuhrer, 1996; Laman & Lankhorst, 1994; Pope & Tarlov, 1991; Wyller, 1997), or are implicit in QOL aphasia research (Lyon et al., 1997; McIntosh, 1997; Ross & Wertz, 2001; Sarno, 1997). Using these models, innovative concepts from leading QOL researchers (Felce & Perry, 1995; Fuhrer, Rintala, Hart, Cleaman, & Young, 1992; Tate, Dijkers, & Johnson-Greene, 1996; World Health Organisation, 1997; Wyller, 1997), and the above findings from stroke and aphasia literature, an operational model was designed for this study (see Figure 1).

The proposed model is modular in construction as it evaluates impairment, activity, participation, and QOL as four separate entities. It represents a comprehensive view of communication in HRQOL and psychological well-being for people with aphasia. The overall concept for this study was that QOL was the collective life experience of people with aphasia, and may be affected by the health condition of a stroke, in the clinical dimensions of language and sensory functioning, communicative activity and ability, and social participation. QOL is described as physical, social, and mental health, and psychological well-being, and was evaluated in terms of its association with emotional

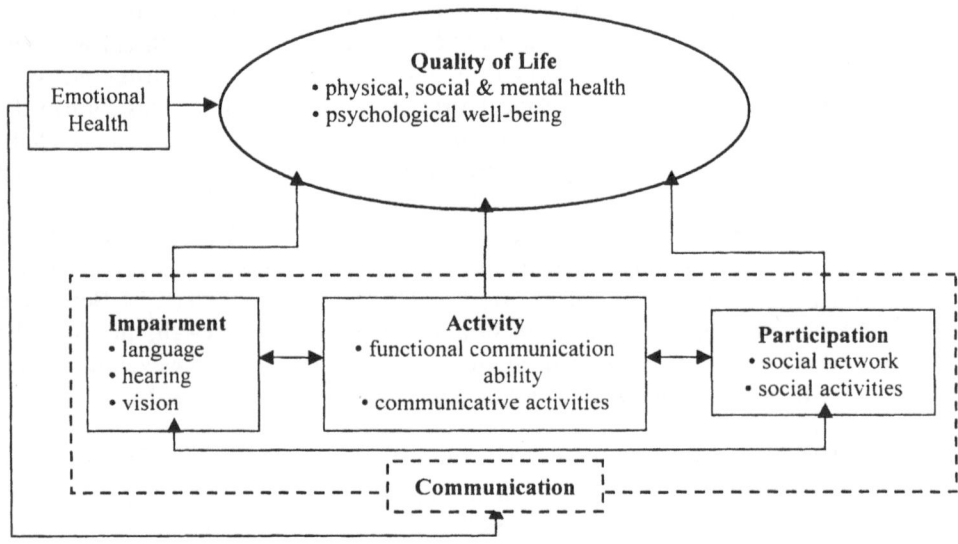

Figure 1. Conceptual and operational model of communication and QOL for people with aphasia.

health, language, vision and hearing impairments, communicative ability and activity, social network relationships, and social activities.

Subsequently, the aim of this study was to investigate the relationships between measures of impairment, activity, and participation, and measures of QOL in people with aphasia, for the purpose of: (1) determining which specific communication assessments were most predictive of QOL; and (2) determining whether HRQOL or psychological well-being was represented more in relationships, thus indicating a focus for QOL in aphasia.

METHODS

Participants

A total of 30 people with aphasia were recruited for the study via university aphasia clinics, three metropolitan hospital speech pathology departments, community stroke groups, and a stroke association. These aphasic participants were part of a larger study of communication and QOL investigating healthy (non-neurological) older people and people with aphasia, and their proxies, using combined research methodologies. Inclusion criteria specified that aphasic participants spoke English as a first language; demonstrated aphasia at time of stroke and self-reported ongoing aphasic difficulties; had reliable yes/no response (no less than 16/20 on WAB Yes/No Questions, Kertesz, 1982); had moderate comprehension at time of interviewing (no less than 5/10 on WAB Comprehension subtest); had no concomitant neurological disease; had normal to moderate mobility (participants requiring a wheelchair were excluded); were 12 months post-stroke;[1] and were living independently in the community.[2]

Demographic and additional information of the 16 female and 14 male aphasic participants are listed in Table 1. The sample was largely fluent, with good auditory com-

---

[1] One participant was marginally less than 12 months post-strike.

[2] Three female participants lived independently in retirement villages (two were frequently active outside the village).

TABLE 1
Demographic and aphasic impairment participant details, $N = 30$

Variable	Mean	Standard deviation	Range
Age	70.7 years	8.4 years	57–88
Education	10.7 years	3.9 years	6–20
Time post-stroke	41 months	25.6 months	10–108
Aphasia quotient	74.4	18.6	21.9–95.8
Spontaneous	15	4.2	4–20
Speech comprehension	8.5	1.3	6–10
Repetition	6.9	2.9	0–10
Naming	6.7	2.4	0–9.5

prehension and average repetition and naming skills, according to performance on Western Aphasia Battery (WAB: Kertesz, 1982). A range of aphasic language profiles was demonstrated: anomic ($n = 15$), conduction ($n = 8$), Broca's ($n = 3$), Wernicke's ($n = 3$), and transcortical sensory (n = 1).

Assessment battery

The test battery included assessments from speech pathology, audiology, optometry, community health, medicine, and psychology. Assessments from these fields were used to evaluate participants' language, hearing, vision, communicative ability and activities, social networks and activities, HRQOL, psychological well-being, and emotional health/ depression. Figure 2 shows the assessments for each section of the model, and each is described below.

(1) Abbreviated version of *Geriatric Depression Scale* (GDS: Sheikh & Yesavage, 1986). Participants responded "yes" or "no" to 15 questions about how they felt over the past week. Scores indicate normal emotional states, mild depression, or moderate to severe depression. The GDS has good reliability, validity, sensitivity, and specificity for older people (McDowell & Newell, 1996). Raw scores were used.

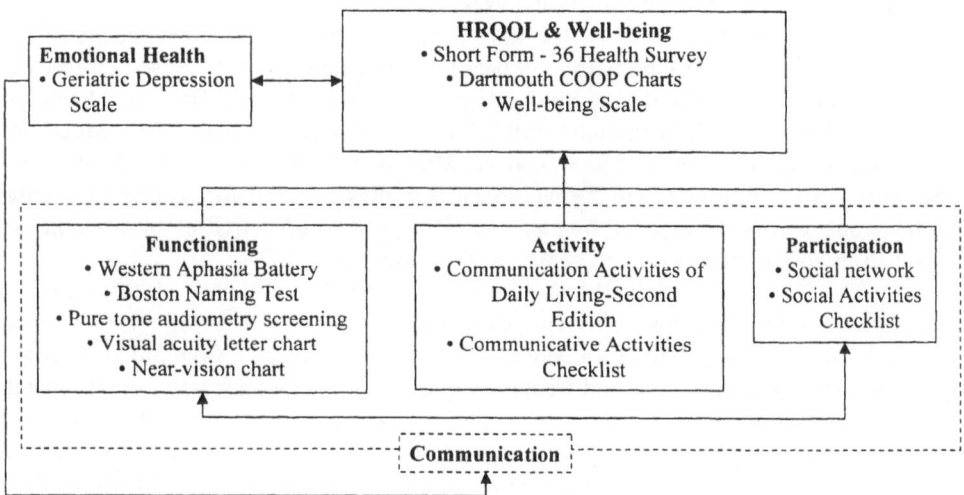

Figure 2. Diagrammatic representation of assessment battery using proposed framework.

(2) *Western Aphasia Battery* (WAB: Kertesz, 1982). Participants completed Aphasia Quotient sections to determine type and severity of language impairment.

(3) The abbreviated 15-item version of *Boston Naming Test* (BNT: Mack, Freed, White Williams, & Henderson, 1992) was used as a clinical assessment of word retrieval difficulties. This version has high reliability and validity with the original 60-item BNT (Kaplan, Goodglass, & Weintraub, 1983).

(4) *Pure tone audiometry* assessed participants' hearing functioning, using air conduction testing at 500, 1000, 2000, and 4000 Hz in both ears. A better-ear average score was used in final statistical analysis.

(5) *Visual acuity letter chart* (Bailey & Lovie, 1976). An 80cm high and 75cm wide white matt card tested distance vision.

(6) *Near-vision chart* (Bailey & Lovie, 1980). An unrelated word sequence, arranged in logarithmic progression of size, evaluated participants' adjusted near vision (with glasses).

(7) *Communication Activities of Daily Living—Second Edition* (CADL-2: Holland, Frattali, & Fromm, 1999). This evaluated participants' functional communication ability through direct observation. Five items were altered for cultural and environmental relevancy for Australian participants. Raw scores out of 100 were used in statistical analysis.

(8) The *Communicative Activities Checklist* (COMACT: Cruice, 2001), specifically designed for the study, measured the frequency and range of activity involvement. This tool was based on numerous sources of related research (Davidson, Worrall, & Hickson, 1998; Le Dorze & Brassard, 1995; Le Dorze, Julien, Brassard, Durocher, & Boivin, 1994; Oxenham, Sheard, & Adams, 1995; Parr, 1995; Stephens & Hetu, 1991; Stephens & Zhao, 1996), as well as item content of the ASHA-FACS (Frattali, Thompson, Holland, Wohl, & Ferketic, 1995), CETI (Lomas, Pickard, & Mohide, 1987), and the Functional Communication Therapy Planner (Worrall, 1999). A total of 45 transactional communicative activities were compiled across speaking/conversation, hearing/listening, reading, and writing. The number of activities that people are involved in comprises the overall score for this assessment.

(9) *Social Network Analysis* (Antonucci & Akiyama, 1987) recorded the number and types of participants' social relationships. The total number of people recorded in a social network was used in final statistical analyses.

(10) *Social Activities Checklist* (SOCACT: Cruice, 2001). This collected range and frequency of social activity participation data for aphasic participants. Based on research and questionnaires within stroke, gerontology, and mental health (Bowling, Farquhar, Grundy, & Formby, 1993; Cummins, 1997; Labi, Phillips, & Gresham, 1980; McDowell & Newell, 1996; Niemi et al., 1988; Reitzes, Mutran, & Verrill, 1995), the 20-item tool measures leisure, informal, and formal social activities checked for regular or average participation across a range of frequencies. The number of activities that people are involved in comprises the overall score for this assessment.

(11) The *Short-Form-36 Health Survey* (SF-36: Ware & Sherbourne, 1992) measured HRQOL in eight subscales across physical and mental health, using the Australian validated version (IQOLA SF-36 Standard Australian Version 1.0). Containing 36 yes/no questions, true/false questions, and frequency questions, this tool generates eight separate subscale scores, which are re-calibrated and transformed producing scores from 0 to 100. Its validity, reliability, responsiveness, and internal consistency are well reported with general elderly populations (Dixon, Heaton, Long, & Warburton, 1994; Garratt, Ruta, Abdalla, Buckingham, & Russell, 1993; Jenkinson, Wright, & Coulter, 1994).

(12) The *Dartmouth COOP Charts* (Nelson et al., 1987) also measured HRQOL in nine charts of functional status through assessment of biological, physical, emotional, and social well-being, and QOL. Each chart poses a single question, and is illustrated with a 5-point response scale, including written description, picture presentation, and numbers. Originally designed to screen patients in primary care, the tool has great potential for aphasic participants because of its illustrations. It generates nine individual chart scores, ranging from 1 to 5. Reliability and validity is reputedly good (Nelson, Landgraf, Hays, Wasson, & Kirk, 1990).

(13) The *"How I Feel About Myself"* Well-being Scale (Thelander, Hoen, & Worsley, 1994) is the condensed version of the short form of the Ryff Psychological Well-being Scale (Ryff, 1989), that was designed by Thelander and colleagues at the York-Durham Aphasia Centre, Ontario. The 24 statements measure six areas of self-acceptance, environmental mastery, autonomy, personal growth, positive relations, and purpose in life as subscales. Participants indicated agreement on a 5-point scale, and numerical values of 1 to 5 were assigned to the response points to generate overall and subscale scores. The original scale is psychometrically sound, and Hoen and colleagues (1997) report adequate reliability and validity on five of their six new scales.

Procedure

Testing was conducted in participants' homes over three to four sessions to reduce fatigue effects, with a maximum of 2 hours per session. QOL and communication were evaluated within a 2-week time-period. QOL assessments were administered first, as communication assessment could raise the awareness of deficit through the nature of testing. QOL assessments and communication assessments were presented in random order, and were administered by a speech pathologist.

QOL questionnaires were administered in interview method, presented in a booklet form, and also read aloud to participants. A cueing or prompting procedure for QOL assessments was developed through pilot testing. Modifications were made to a number of assessments. For example, true/false questions (SF-36) and statements (well-being scale) were changed to yes/no questions for some participants. On distance and near vision tests, some participants wrote the letters that they could see, or pointed to letters in a random alphabet string, instead of reporting aloud.

Analysis

Data were analysed using exploratory data plots, Pearson's product–moment r correlations, and linear and non-linear (b-spline) regression coefficients. Once predictors (communication variables) of the dependent (QOL) variable had been identified, they were placed in a maximal multiple regression model. The best predictors were chosen by stepwise regression with backward elimination, wherein uninformative terms were dropped on the basis of their Akaike's Information Criteria (AIC: Chambers & Hastie, 1992). (The AIC assesses the benefit–penalty of including each term. The benefit is the reduction in error, the penalty is the increase in the complexity of the model. If removal of a term reduces the AIC, it is deleted from the model.) This statistical modelling technique was used consistently, and systematically determined the relative strength of numerous predictor variables. Final models, corrected for confounding variables, revealed the strongest predictors, and the variance (or deviance from categorical data and ordinal regression) have been reported. Different regression models were dependent on the data—Gaussian or Poisson for normal data, binomial for COMACT and SOCACT data, and ordinal for COOP charts data.

RESULTS

Revised briefly, the aim of this study was to investigate the strength of association between communication assessments (i.e., impairment, activity, and participation level assessments) and QOL assessments (HRQOL and well-being). The objectives were: (1) to determine which specific communication assessments were most predictive of QOL; and (2) to determine whether HRQOL or psychological well-being was represented more in relationships, indicating a focus for QOL in aphasia.

Descriptive communication and QOL results

Participants had mild to moderate–severe aphasia, with more than half the sample having impaired naming (BNT) and hearing functioning, and approximately half the sample having impaired distance and near vision functioning. Participants' sensory impairments (hearing and vision) were predominantly mild in degree. Participants' CADL-2 scores showed a range of moderately low to high functional communication ability (range = 31–95). A restricted range of communicative activities was noted, with participants frequently involved in listening activities, and very infrequently involved in reading and writing activities. Participants named a range of social network contacts (mean = 21, SD = 12.7, range = 5–51), however they were only involved in a small number of social activities, especially leisure activities.

SF-36 data were skewed towards the maximum end of range scores for five of the eight subscale scores (i.e., Role Physical, Body Pain, Social Functioning, Role Emotional, and Mental Health). Results indicated the sample had reasonable social functioning, freedom from body pain, and good mental health, but poor physical functioning and vitality. Likewise, COOP data were skewed towards the maximum end of range scores for seven of the nine charts (i.e., Feelings, Daily Activities, Social Activities, Pain, Overall Health, Social Support, and Quality of Life). Results illustrated high social support, good social activities and little pain, but poor physical fitness. Compared to HRQOL assessments, the well-being scale and subscales demonstrated relatively more normal distributions of scores. Participants indicated greatest autonomy (control over self) but poorest environmental mastery (control over environment and living situation). Of the participants, 26 had normal emotional health on the GDS, 6 presented with mild depressive symptoms, and the remaining 3 scored as moderately to severely depressed.

Influential demographic variables (age, educational level, time post-stroke, emotional health score) were investigated for their impact on participants' communication and QOL. Overall, age affected communication, and emotional health affected QOL. Older age correlated with greater near vision impairment ($r = .6$, $p = .001$), greater hearing impairment ($r = .44$, $p = .02$), lower functional communication ability ($r = -.6$, $p = .001$), involvement in fewer communicative activities ($r = -.5$, $p = .01$), and participation in fewer social activities ($r = -.4$, $p < .05$). Better emotional health correlated strongly with better HRQOL and higher psychological well-being scores across many variables of QOL at the $p = .005$ level (Table 2).

Model for communication and the SF-36

Exploratory data plots and Pearson's r correlations revealed that near vision, CADL-2,

TABLE 2
Significant Pearson *r* correlations between emotional health and QOL of participants, *N* = 30

SF-36 subscales	COOP Charts	Well-being Scale & subscale
Physical functioning −.6	Social activities −.8	Total scale −.7
Role physical −.6	Quality of life −.5	Environmental mastery −.6
General health .8		Purpose in life −.6
Vitality −.6		Self acceptance −.7
Social functioning −.7		
Mental healt −.6		

number of social activities, and emotional health correlated with SF-36 subscales. Outlier data from two participants on near and distance vision were removed from the analysis. Linear regressions demonstrated that demographic variables entirely predicted scores on two subscales: better emotional health predicted more Vitality (regression coefficient $r = -3.26, p = .003; r^2 = .29$); and a combination of emotional health ($-3.43, p = .002; r^2 = .27$) and younger age ($1.9, p = .06, r^2 = .09$) predicted better Mental Health.

Figure 3 illustrates only significant relationships between communication variables and SF-36 subscales. Regression coefficients (r) are not represented in the figure, but instead are tabulated in Appendix 1. Variance (r^2 = between 0 and 1) is reported on the figure alongside each predictor, to illustrate their relative strength in prediction. Stepwise regressions on General Health and Social Functioning demonstrated that emotional health and near vision were the strongest predictors, and overpowered the associations of Social Activities and CADL-2, respectively. Emotional health was significantly related to HRQOL, and influenced every relationship in the figure. The links suggest that poor daily physical ability and general health determined participant social activities. Better near vision and functional communication ability predicted better social functioning. The stepwise regressions demonstrated that near vision impairment was stronger than activity and participation variables. The association between better near vision and better general health and physical functioning, indicates that near vision may be operating as an index of physiological age in the sample.

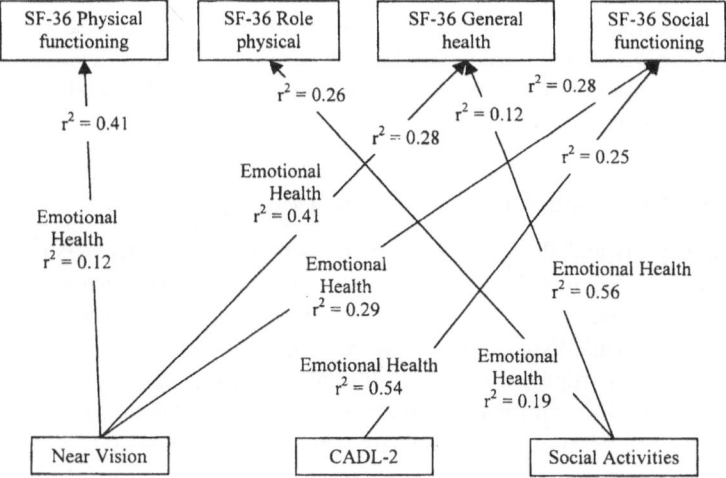

Figure 3. Significant relationships between impairment, activity, and participation and SF-36, *N* = 30.

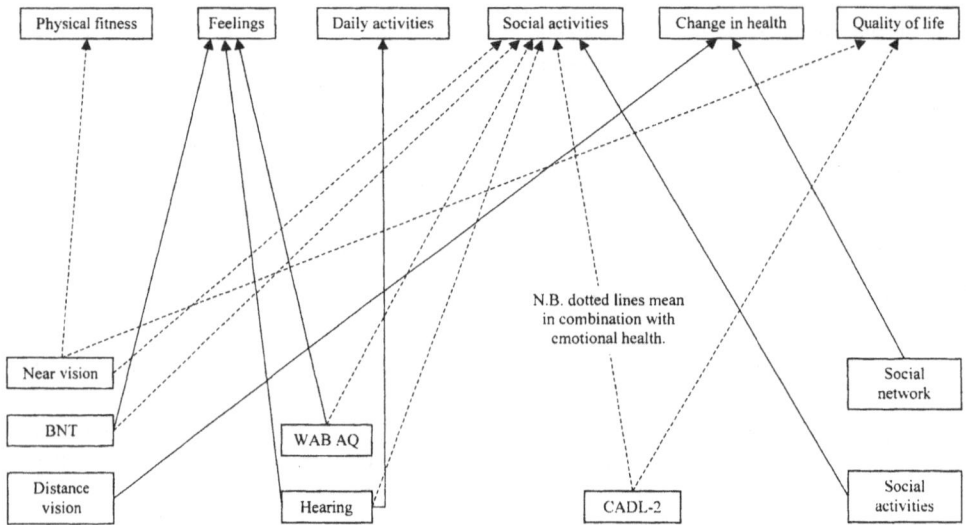

Figure 4.   Significant relationships between impairment, activity, participation, and the COOP Charts, $N = 30$.

Model for communication and the Dartmouth COOP charts

Exploratory data plots and Pearson's *r* correlations revealed that all communication variables, excluding communicative activities, were possibly associated with the nine COOP charts. Because of the ordinal nature of COOP data, ordinal regression analysis was used, which precludes modelling more than one variable in the same regression, and variance is not reported. Categories four and five on the Physical Fitness chart were collapsed, and categories one and two on Quality of Life also, because of small participant numbers.

Figure 4 presents only significant relationships between communication variables and COOP charts. Regression coefficients are tabulated in Appendix 1. Emotional health and communication at all three levels related to a considerable number of charts, specifically COOP Social Activities. In summary, better language functioning, better functional communication abilities, and more social activities were positively associated with better social health, emotional health, and QOL. Language and hearing predicted emotional health (COOP Feelings), and participants' health determined social networks. Similar to SF-36 findings, better near vision was associated with COOP Social Activities, and distance vision related to Health.

Model for communication and the Well-being scale

Exploratory data plots and Pearson's *r* correlations revealed that near vision, WAB AQ, WAB spontaneous speech, CADL-2, social network, number of leisure activities, age, and emotional health were associated with participant well-being. Outlier data from two participants in near and distance vision were removed from the analysis. Emotional health only predicted participant scores on Purpose in Life (-3.95, $p = .000$; $r^2 = .36$).

Figure 5 illustrates the significant relationships between communication variables and well-being scales. Regression coefficients are tabulated in Appendix 1. Participants with better near vision had more autonomy, environmental mastery, and total well-being. Participants with more environmental mastery also had larger social networks. Better

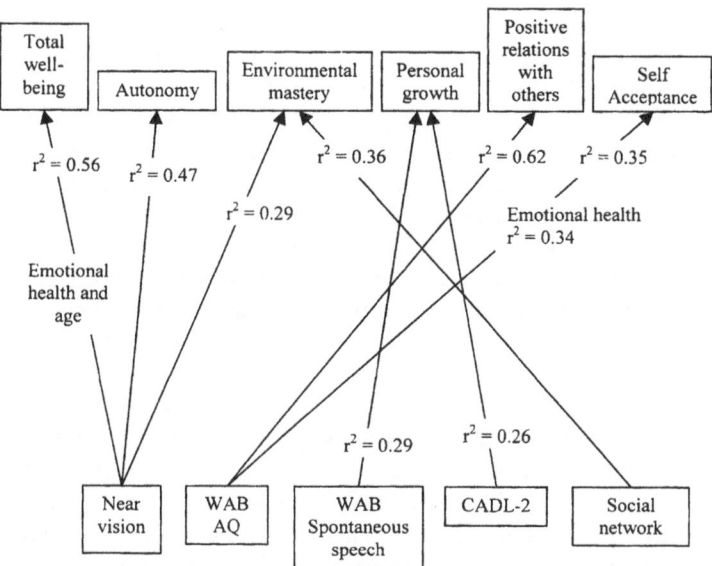

Figure 5.   Significant relationships between impairment, activity, participation, and the Well-being Scale, $N = 30$.

language functioning, and functional communication ability predicted higher personal development, more positive social relations with others and self-acceptance. According to the subscales' definition (Hoen et al., 1997), these findings suggest that language contributes to life "fulfilment" whereas near vision contributes to "independence" in psychological well-being.

DISCUSSION

This research sought to address the need for greater knowledge regarding the relationships among communication impairment, activity, participation, well-being, and QOL (McNeil, 2001). This study confirms that communication is strongly associated with social HRQOL and psychological well-being for people with aphasia. Participants with higher functioning and better communication ability had fewer social functioning limitations, higher QOL, higher emotional health, and higher personal, relational, and self-acceptance well-being.

In terms of the operational model, functional communication ability (CADL-2) was consistently represented in all three QOL results models. There were also more associations between the CADL-2 and QOL subscales, than between impairment assessments and QOL subscales. This indicates that communication ability at the activity level CADL-2 was most predictive of participants' QOL. It is also important to note that impairment assessments had strong predictive powers determining QOL.

These findings empirically support the theoretically debated emotional, social, and psychological issues of patients with aphasia (Gainotti, 1997), and concur with other research demonstrating similar links between impairment, communication ability, and psychosocial well-being in individuals with aphasia (Boles, 1997). Evidence from this research indicates that communication and communication disability at the activity level is associated with social activities, social networks, social support, and positive relationships with other people. Both language and social activities contributed to personal growth and development, and self-acceptance. These current findings concur with the reports of people with aphasia and their family and friends regarding how aphasic communication difficulties have impacted on their social lives and their person (Jordan & Kaiser, 1996; Le Dorze & Brassard, 1995; Parr, Byng, Gilpin, & Ireland, 1997; Zemva, 1999). Aphasic participants' language functioning was also important to their own well-being, namely personal growth, positive relationships with others, and self-acceptance subscales. Thus, the current research supports the conjecture made by Brumfitt (1993) that language is linked to the growth and acceptance of self.

Findings illustrated that impairments other than communication, namely to hearing and vision, also predicted social health, and are important to identify. Sensory impairments can exacerbate the effects of other impairments on disability (Kempen, Verbrugge, Merrill, & Ormel, 1998). The current results concur with the literature on the impact of sensory functioning on older people's activities (Carabellese et al., 1993; Clark, Bond, & Sanchez, 1999; Hickson & Worrall, 1997, Resnick, Fries, & Verbrugge, 1997; Scott, Smiddy, Schiffman, Feuer, & Pappas, 1999; Stephens & Zhao, 1996). However, a triangular relationship between vision (impairment), physical and general health (HRQOL), and social activities and networks (participation) suggests that participants' physiological health was a hidden confounding variable. This complex association has previously been reported in stroke patients (Wade, Legh-Smith, & Langton-Hewer, 1985) and healthy older people (Mendes de Leon, Glass, Beckett, Seeman, Evans, & Berkman, 1999; Unger, McAvay, Bruce, Berkman, & Seeman, 1999).

This study highlighted that factors other than aphasia determined people's participation and QOL, and as Lamb (1996) noted, emotional and functional limitations often co-occur and correlate with lower QOL. Post-stroke depression, affecting up to 70% of people (Sarno, 1993), is an important variable for consideration when evaluating QOL for people with aphasia (Code, Hemsley, & Hermann, 1999). Emotional and physical health are important for people with aphasia as both reduce the opportunities for communication in social interactions and thus reduce QOL. Comprehensive evaluation and consideration in communication intervention is implicated.

Two cautionary notes are made regarding the prediction of QOL and the purpose of QOL assessment in clinical rehabilitation. First, QOL and the elements associated with it are dynamic in nature. Felce and Perry (1995) noted that "knowledge of one set cannot predict another because the relationships between them may not remain constant ... and the elements that define QOL are all open to external influence" (p. 63). Therefore, despite the evidence of this research for the relationships between communication and QOL, the associations are not likely to be the same for different groups of people with aphasia, or even for the same people over time. Consequently, there is a need to assess at all levels of impairment, activity, and participation, despite the predictive powers demonstrated by functional communication ability and overall language functioning in people with aphasia.

Second, clinicians must be cautious as to the purpose and use of QOL scores in outcome measurement. QOL is highly applicable in rehabilitation as a means of ensuring individually relevant rehabilitation, and is useful for measuring individual progress. Given that QOL research is relatively new in speech pathology, it cannot yet be used for group or service level decision-making processes. QOL evaluation in aphasia has several methodological, reliability, and validity problems. Evidence from previous research (Cruice, Hirsch, Worrall, Holland, & Hickson, 2000) has demonstrated that: existing QOL assessments require modification for people with aphasia; the reliability of modified versions is unknown; and communication and social relationships are insufficiently represented in assessments. Ongoing research into these issues is providing some much-needed greater knowledge about QOL evaluation with people with aphasia (Hilari & Byng, 2001).

Clinical implications

The research provides strong evidence for addressing QOL in rehabilitation for people with aphasia. Clearly language functioning (impairment), functional communication ability (activity), emotional and social health, and psychological well-being, are important for improving clients' QOL. This study illustrates how these five elements are interrelated, and the findings suggest two approaches in intervention: indirect (working on communication) and/or direct (working on social health and psychological well-being). Some specific directions for therapy goals, treatment techniques, and approaches to aphasia therapy are suggested below.

Byng, Pound and Parr (2000) proposed six goals for aphasia intervention: enhancing communication; identifying and dismantling barriers to social participation; adaptation of identity; promoting a healthy psychological state; promotion of autonomy and choice; and health promotion/illness prevention. The current findings can be juxtaposed against many of their goals. For example, the focus on emotional health and psychological well-being in the current study, may be understood as three goals of adaptation of identity, promotion of healthy psychological state, and promotion of autonomy and choice. Their chapter, "Living with aphasia: A framework for therapy interventions" (Byng et al., 2000), outlines a range of intervention programmes aimed at addressing these goals. Using the example above, potential interventions may include involving the person with aphasia in a self-advocacy project group, or offering educational packages to other services about aphasia. Intervention may also dismantle barriers in the process, such as changing the way written materials are provided, thus enabling the person with aphasia to access and understand information, and make his/her own decisions.

The current research findings indicate that assessment at the activity level is highly pertinent for people with aphasia, and imply that therapies should be principally aimed at improving functional communication and reducing activity limitations. Speech pathologists can work on a person's daily communication abilities by focusing on real-life activities, often using a total communication approach. Instruments such as the *Functional Communication Therapy Planner* (Worrall, 1999) are useful in delineating the process of identifying functional goals and activities with clients. Pound, Parr, Lindsay, and Woolf (2000) in their latest book *Beyond Aphasia* give many examples of total communication in therapeutic activities.

Reducing activity limitations also often involves training family and friends of people with aphasia in methods that facilitate the communicative interaction (Rogers, Alarcon, & Olswang, 1999). An example of such is the programme *Supported Conversation for Adults with Aphasia* (Kagan, Black, Duchan, Simmons-Mackie, & Square, 2001). Two further landmark studies illustrate how important effective conversation is between people with aphasia and their communication partners. They also indicate that working at the activity level can also have spillover effects into other areas of participation and QOL. Lyon and colleagues (1997) used such *Communication Partners* for teaching effective communication between pairs of people. It resulted in pronounced positive effects on people's involvement in new activities, and fostered more community integration and interaction. Similarly, *Conversation Partners Therapy* had significant positive effects across impairment, communication abilities, and well-being in individuals with aphasia (Boles, 1997). Functional communication also has immediate relevance to people with aphasia as communicative situations are often socially framed (Lomas et al., 1987). Language impairment was also an important predictor of emotional health, social activities, relationships with others, and self-acceptance. Therefore, any treatment approach that improves language is relevant to improving people's QOL. As the literature abounds in treatments for aphasia, none is specified here. Treatments that improve functional communication and reduce language impairment are ideal.

Transparently important in the model was the value of social health, therefore intervention that is undertaken in groups adds a social frame of reference. Group work with people with aphasia has gained momentum over the past decade and has proved efficacious (Elman & Berstein-Ellis, 1999). Group communication treatment has documented the psychosocial benefits for people with aphasia, such as being with others, making friends, having the support of others, and being able to help others (Elman & Berstein-Ellis, 1999). Groups may be language and communication focused (Avent, 1997), or discussion or recreation focused (Drummond & Walker, 1996; Marshall, 1999; Sarno, 1997). Group work may also provide a level of social support, an important variable for managing depressive symptoms (King, Shade-Zeldow, Carlson, Feldman, & Phillip, 2002).

The emotional health of people with aphasia clearly warrants much attention in rehabilitation. Referral to other professionals for counselling and support is necessary. Counselling that focuses on adaptation can bring about an understanding of purpose in life, which leads to growth and self-actualisation (Clarke, 1998). In addition, speech pathologists need to broaden their own intervention to include assessment of emotional health, treatment of psychosocial issues (Müller, 1999), and supportive therapy approaches that facilitate healthy emotional states. Facilitated story telling (Ronnberg, 1998) and narrative therapies may be relevant, as they incidentally address several communication levels but more importantly foster personal development and self-acceptance in psychological well-being. Byng and colleagues (2000) provide several suggestions for adapting and creating new identities, such as personal portfolios, counselling, and creative arts groups.

Supportive therapy approaches, which facilitate healthy emotional and psychological states, relate not only to what clinicians do in the way of therapy (as above), but also to how they do it and who they are. Jordan and Kaiser (1996) indicate that speech pathologists should act as resources for clients by supporting and enabling clients, and sharing expertise and knowledge, rather than being experts who dominate and manage disabled clients. The former approach in therapeutic interactions promotes an environment for client autonomy and choice, and is suggested for QOL-focused rehabilitation. QOL focus also involves personalising aphasia in the context of each client.

A new communication-related quality of life model in aphasia

A revised version of the operational model (Figure 1) is proposed as a new communication-related QOL (CRQOL) model (see Figure 6). It is apparent that communication is not a determinant of HRQOL, which is commonly understood to be physical health, and thus, a generic HRQOL focus is inappropriate for people with aphasia. However, communication was associated with social health indices of the SF-36 and COOP charts, indicating that this dimension of health is relevant for people with communication disability. Thus QOL could be more appropriately conceptualised as social health and psychological well-being. In the CRQOL model, communication is again conceptualised

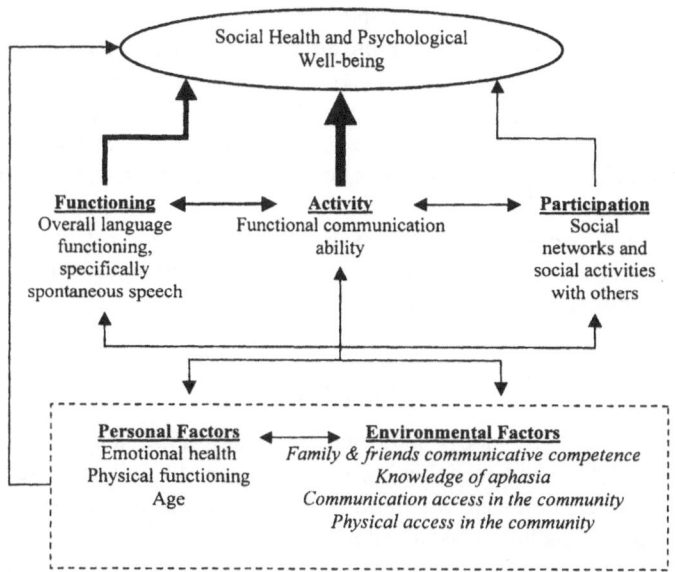

Figure 6.   A new communication-related quality of life (CRQOL) model for people with aphasia.

as the three dimensions of functioning, activity, and participation, using the ICIDH-2 framework. The ICIDH-2 framework is maintained in the model because: (1) it is a widely understood and accepted framework used by aphasia researchers and clinicians (Eadie, 2001; Enderby, 1992; Frattali, 1998; Le Dorze & Brassard, 1995; Oxenham et al., 1995; Rogers et al., 1999); and (2) it assists with interprofessional relations, as it is used internationally for description and data collection, regarding the consequences of a range of health conditions.

The current research supports the communication indicators that were chosen in the initial model (Figure 1) for impairment and activity. There was considerable overlap between the social participation indicators (social network and activities) and social HRQOL components (social functioning and activities), highlighting the blurred boundary between participation and QOL. Difficulty in separating these two concepts in speech pathology has been noted before (Hirsch & Holland, 2000). These findings pose the challenge of whether to define a new concept of participation for people with aphasia (leaving social health as part of QOL), or whether to subsume social health as participation (leaving psychological well-being as the sole interpretation of QOL). Further research is required to determine how aphasia impacts on people's participation, and thus what construct of participation is valid and appropriate.

The study's findings suggest that personal contextual factors, namely emotional health, physiological and/or physical functioning, and age, influenced aphasia participants' communication and QOL. As such, they have been incorporated into the new CRQOL model. Other current research in aphasia suggests that variables beyond the person with aphasia impact on their communication experience and QOL, such as the communicative competence of family and friends, knowledge of aphasia, and communication and physical access in the community (Byng et al., 2000; Code et al., 2001; Kagan et al., 2001). These issues have been integrated in Figure 6 as italicised environmental contextual factors.

Documenting the personal and environmental factors enables clinicians to justify wide-ranging intervention for people with aphasia that goes beyond improving clients' language and communication. Some examples of the scope of aphasia rehabilitation are: (1) training family and friends' communicative competence; (2) improving aphasic people's emotional health; and (3) devising projects to address physical community barriers to participation. Communication rehabilitation that strategically addresses personal and environmental factors, complements a language and communication focus. In summary, the findings suggest that communication (functioning, activity, participation) and context (personal and environmental factors) are equally important, as well as interdependent, for the person with aphasia. Furthermore, it is most likely that personal and environmental contextual factors are likewise interdependent, a finding that has not previously been recognised in the ICIDH-2.

CONCLUSION

Speech pathologists are ultimately interested in determining the impact of people's communication on QOL, and in doing so, justifying our discipline's intervention. Previously, QOL has been perceived as a multi-factorial concept in rehabilitation, making it impossible for speech pathologists to address QOL in a profession-specific manner. However, this research provides evidence for clinicians to selectively focus on social health and psychological well-being as QOL for people with aphasia. People's emotional health, language functioning, and functional communication ability are largely predictive of their QOL. Finally, it provides direction for specific choices and approaches to aphasia therapy, based on their greatest potential impact on clients' QOL.

REFERENCES

Ahlsiö, B., Britton, M., Murray, V., & Theorelli, T. (1984). Disablement and quality of life after stroke. *Stroke*, *15*(5), 886–890.

Antonucci, T. C., & Akiyama, H. (1987). Social networks in adult life and a preliminary examination of the convoy model. *Journal of Gerontology*, *42*(5), 519–527.

Aström, M., Asplund, K., & Aström, T. (1992). Psychosocial function and life satisfaction after stroke. *Stroke*, *23*, 527–531.

Avent, J. (1997). *Manual of cooperative group treatment for aphasia*. Boston: Butterworth Heinemann.

Bailey, I., & Lovie, J. (1976). New design principles for visual acuity letter charts. *American Journal of Optometry and Physiological Optics*, *53*(11), 740–745.

Bailey, I., & Lovie, J. (1980). The design and use of a new near-vision chart. *American Journal of Optometry and Physiological Optics*, *57*, 378–387.

Bays, C. (2001). Quality of life of stroke survivors: A research synthesis. *Journal of Neuroscience Nursing*, *33*(6), 310–316.

Bech, P. (1993). *Rating scales for psychopathology, health status, and quality of life: A compendium on documentation in accordance with the DSM-III-R and WHO systems*. Berlin: Springer-Verlag.

Bendz, M. (2000). Rules of relevance after a stroke. *Social Science & Medicine*, *51*, 713–723.

Boles, L. (1997). Conversation analysis as a dependent measure in communication therapy with four individuals with aphasia. *Asia Pacific Journal of Speech, Language and Hearing*, *2*, 43–61.

Bowling, A., Farquhar, M., Grundy, E., & Formby, J. (1993). Changes in life satisfaction over a two and a half year period among very elderly people living in London. *Social Science & Medicine*, *36*(5), 641–655.

Brumfitt, S. (1993). Losing your sense of self: What aphasia can do. *Aphasiology*, *7*(6), 569–575.

Brumfitt, S. (1998). The measurement of psychological well-being in the person with aphasia. *International Journal of Language and Communication Disorders*, *33*(Suppl), 116–120.

Buscherhof, J. R. (1998). From abled to disabled: A life transition. *Topics in Stroke Rehabilitation*, *5*(2), 19–29.

Byng, S., Pound, C., & Parr, S. (2000). Living with aphasia: A framework for therapy interventions. In I. Papathanasiou (Ed.), *Acquired neurogenic communication disorders*. London: Whurr Publishers.

Cant, R. (1997). Rehabilitation following stroke: A participant perspective. *Disability and Rehabilitation*, *19*(7), 297–304.

Carabellese, C., Appollonio, I., Rozzini, R., Bianchetti, A., Frisoni, G., Frattola, L., & Trabucchi, M. (1993). Sensory impairment and quality of life in a community elderly population. *Journal of American Geriatrics Society*, *41*, 401–407.

Chambers, J., & Hastie, T. (1992). *Statistical modelling in S*. London: Chapman & Hall.

Clark, M., Bond, M., & Sanchez, L. (1999). The effect of sensory impairment on the lifestyle activities of older people. *Australasian Journal on Ageing*, *18*(3), 124–129.

Clarke, H. (1998). Chapter 5. Harry's story: Becoming a counsellor following a stroke. In D. Syder (Ed.), *Wanting to talk: Counselling case studies in communication disorders* (pp. 105–131). London: Whurr Publishers.

Code, C., Hemsley, G., & Hermann, M. (1999). The emotional impact of aphasia. *Seminars in Speech and Language*, *20*(1), 19–31.

Code, C., Simmons-Mackie, N., Armstrong, E., Stiegler, L., Armstrong, J., Bushby, E., Carew-Price, P., Curtis, H., Haynes, P., McLeod, E., Muhleisen, V., Neate, J., Nikolas, A., Rolfe, D. Rubly, C., Simpson, R., & Webber, A. (2001). The public awareness of aphasia: An international survey. *International Journal of Language and Communication Disorders*, *36*(Suppl), 1–6.

Cruice, M. (2001). *Communication and quality of life in older people with aphasia and healthy older people*. Unpublished doctoral thesis: Department of Speech Pathology and Audiology, University of Queensland.

Cruice, M., Hirsch, F., Worrall, L., Holland, A., & Hickson, L. (2000). Quality of life for people with aphasia: Performance on and usability of quality of life assessments. *Asia Pacific Journal of Speech, Language and Hearing*, *5*, 85–91.

Cruice, M., Worrall, L., & Hickson, L. (2000). Quality-of-life measurement in speech pathology and audiology. *Asia Pacific Journal of Speech, Language and Hearing*, *5*, 1–20.

Cummins, R. (1997). *Comprehensive Quality of Life Scale – Intellectual/Cognitive Disability* (5th Ed.). Melbourne: Deakin University, School of Psychology.

Davidson, B., Worrall, L., & Hickson, L. (1998). *Observed communication activities of people with aphasia and healthy older people*. Paper presented at the 8th International Aphasia Rehabilitation conference, Kwa Maritane, South Africa, August.

Dixon, P., Heaton, J., Long, A., & Warburton, A. (1994). Reviewing and applying the SF-36. *Outcomes Briefing*, *4*(August), 3–20.

Drummond, A., & Walker, M. (1996). Generalisation of the effects of leisure rehabilitation for stroke patients. *British Journal of Occupational Therapy*, *59*(7), 330–334.

Eadie, T. (2001). The ICIDH-2: Theoretical and clinical implications for speech-language pathology. *Journal of Speech Language Pathology and Audiology*, *25*(4), 181–200.

Elman, R., & Berstein-Ellis, E. (1999). Psychosocial aspects of group communication treatment: Preliminary findings. *Seminars in Speech and Language*, *20*(1), 65–83.

Enderby, P. (1992). Outcome measures in speech therapy: Impairment, disability, handicap and distress. *Health Trends*, *24*(2), 61–64.

Engell, B., Huber, W., & Hütter, B. (1998). *Quality of life measurement in aphasic patients*. Proceedings of the 24th International Association of Logopaedics and Phoniatrics Congress, August, Amsterdam.

Felce, D., & Perry, J. (1995). Quality of life: Its definition and measurement. *Research in Developmental Disabilities*, *16*(1), 51–74.

Frattali, C., Thompson, C., Holland, A., Wohl, C., & Ferketic, M. (1995). *American Speech-Language-Hearing Association: Functional Assessment of Communication Skills for Adults (ASHA-FACS)*. Rockville, MD: American Speech-Language-Hearing Association.

Frattali, C. M. (1998). *Measuring outcomes in speech-language pathology*. New York: Thieme.

Fuhrer, M. J. (1996). The subjective well-being of people with spinal cord injury: Relationships to impairment, disability, and handicap. *Topics in Spinal Cord Injury Rehabilitation*, *1*(4), 56–71.

Fuhrer, M. J., Rintala, D. H., Hart, K. A., Cleaman, R., & Young, M. E. (1992). Relationship of life satisfaction to impairment, disability and handicap among persons with spinal cord injury living in the community. *Archives of Physical and Medical Rehabilitation*, *73*, 552–557.

Gainotti, G. (1997). Emotional, psychological and psychosocial problems of aphasic patients: An introduction. *Aphasiology*, *11*(7), 635–650.

Garratt, A. M., Ruta, D. A., Abdalla, M. I., Buckingham, J. K., & Russell, I. T. (1993). The SF-36 health survey questionnaire: An outcome measure suitable for routine use within the NHS? *British Medical Journal*, *306*, 1440–1444.

Hemsley, G., & Code, C. (1996). Interactions between recovery in aphasia, emotional and psychosocial factors in subjects with aphasia, their significant others and speech pathologists. *Disability and Rehabilitation*, *18*(11), 567–584.

Hickson, L., & Worrall, L. (1997). Hearing impairment, disability and handicap in older people. *Critical Reviews in Physical and Rehabilitation Medicine, 9*(3&4), 219–243.

Hilari, K., & Byng, S. (2001). Measuring quality of life in people with aphasia: The Stroke Specific Quality of Life Scale. *International Journal of Human Communication Disorders, 36*(Suppl), 86–91.

Hinckley, J. J. (1998). Investigating the predictors of lifestyle satisfaction among younger adults with chronic aphasia. *Aphasiology, 12*(7/8), 509–518.

Hirsch, F., & Holland, A. (2000). Beyond activity: Measuring participation in society and quality of life. In L. Worrall & C. Frattali (Eds.), *Neurogenic communication disorders: A functional approach* (pp. 35–54). New York: Thieme.

Hoen, B., Thelander, M., & Worsley, J. (1997). Improvement in psychological well-being of people with aphasia and their families: Evaluation of a community-based programme. *Aphasiology, 11*(7), 681–691.

Holland, A., Frattali, C., & Fromm, D. (1999). *Communication Activities of Daily Living – Second Edition.* Texas: Pro-Ed.

Jenkinson, C., Wright, L., & Coulter, A. (1994). Criterion validity and reliability of the SF-36 in a population sample. *Quality of Life Research, 3*, 7–12.

Jordan, L., & Kaiser, W. (1996). *Aphasia: A social approach.* London: Chapman & Hall.

Kagan, A., Black, S., Duchan, J., Simmons-Mackie, N., & Square, P. (2001). Training volunteers as conversation partners using "supported conversation for adults with aphasia" (SCA): A controlled trial. *Journal of Speech, Language, and Hearing Research, 44*(3), 624–638

Kaplan, E., Goodglass, H., & Weintraub, S. (1983). *Boston Naming Test (Revised).* Philadelphia, PA: Lea & Febiger.

Kappelle, L. J., Adams, H. P., Heffner, M. L., Torner, J. C., Gomez, F., & Biller, J. (1994). Prognosis of young adults with ischemic stroke: A long-term follow-up study assessing recurrent vascular events and functional outcome in the Iowa registry of stroke in young adults. *Stroke, 25*(7), 1360–1365.

Kauhanen, M., Korpelainen, J., Hiltunen, P., Nieminen, P., Sotaniemi, K., & Myllalä, V. (2000). Domains and determinants of quality of life after stroke caused by brain infarction. *Archives of Physical Medicine and Rehabilitation, 81*, 1541–1546.

Kempen, G. I., Verbrugge, L., Merrill, S., & Ormel, J. (1998). The impact of multiple impairments on disability in community-dwelling older people. *Age and Ageing, 27*, 595–604.

Kertesz, A. (1982). *The Western Aphasia Battery.* New York: Grune & Stratton.

King, R., Shade-Zeldow, Y., Carlson, C., Feldman, J., & Phillip, M. (2002). Adaptation to stroke: A longitudinal study of depressive symptoms, physical health, and coping process. *Topics in Stroke Rehabilitation, 9*(1), 46–66.

Labi, M. L., Phillips, T. F., & Gresham, G. E. (1980). Psychosocial disability in physically restored long-term stroke survivors. *Archives of Physical and Medical Rehabilitation, 61*, 561–565.

Laman, H., & Lankhorst, G. J. (1994). Subjective weighting of disability: An approach to quality of life assessment. *Disability and Rehabilitation, 16*(4), 198–204.

Lamb, V. L. (1996). A cross-cultural study of quality of life factors associated with patterns of elderly disablement. *Social Science & Medicine, 42*(3), 363–377.

LaPointe, L. L. (1999). Quality of life with aphasia. *Seminars in Speech and Language, 20*(1), 5–17.

Le Dorze, G., & Brassard, C. (1995). A description of the consequences of aphasia on aphasic persons and their relatives and friends based on the WHO model of chronic diseases. *Aphasiology, 9*(3), 239–255.

Le Dorze, G., Julien, M., Brassard, C., Durocher, J., & Boivin, G. (1994). An analysis of the communication of adult residents of a long-term care hospital as perceived by their caregivers. *European Journal of Disorders of Communication, 29*, 241–267.

Löfgren, B., Gustafson, Y., & Nyberg, L. (1999). Psychological well-being 3 years after severe stroke. *Stroke, 30*, 567–572.

Lomas, J., Pickard, L., & Mohide, A. (1987). Patient versus clinican item generation for quality of life measures: The case of language-disabled adults. *Medical Care, 25*(8), 764–769.

Lyon, J. G., Cariski, D., Keisler, L., Rosenbek, J., Levine, R., Kumpula, J., Ryff, C., Coyne, S., & Blanc, M. (1997). Communication partners: Enhancing participation in life and communication for adults with aphasia in natural settings. *Aphasiology, 11*(7), 693–708.

Mack, W. J., Freed, D. M., White Williams, B., & Henderson, V. W. (1992). Boston Naming Test: Shortened versions for use in Alzheimer's disease. *Journal of Gerontology, 47*(3), 154–158.

Marshall, R. (1999). *Introduction to group treatment for aphasia: Design and management.* Boston: Butterworth Heinemann.

McDowell, I., & Newell, C. (1996). *Measuring health: A guide to rating scales and questionnaires* (2nd Edn.). New York: Oxford University Press.

McIntosh, K. (1997). Analysis of relationships among measures of language impairment, communication disability, social support and quality of life handicap, in late post-onset adult aphasic persons. *Dissertation Abstracts International: Section B: The Sciences and Engineering, 58*(3–B), 1243.

McNeil, M. (2001). Promoting paradigm change: The importance of evidence. *Advances in Speech-Language Pathology, 3*(1), 55–58.

Mendes de Leon, C., Glass, T., Beckett, L., Seeman, T., Evans, D., & Berkman, L. (1999). Social networks and disability transitions across eight intervals of yearly data in the New Haven EPESE. *Journal of Gerontology, 54B*(3), S162–S172.

Müller, D. (1999). Managing psychosocial adjustment to aphasia. *Seminars in Speech and Language, 20*(1), 85–92.

Newborn, B. (1998). Quality of life for long term recovery in stroke. *Topics in Stroke Rehabilitation, 5*(2), 61–63.

Nelson, E., Landgraf, J., Hays, R., Wasson, J., & Kirk, J. (1990). The functional status of patients: How can it be measured in physicians' offices? *Medical Care, 28*(12), 1111–1126.

Nelson, E., Wasson, J., Kirk, J., Keller, A., Clark, D., Dietrich, A., Stewart, A., & Zubkoff, M. (1987). Assessment of function in routine clinical practice: Description of the COOP Chart method and preliminary findings. *Journal of Chronic Disease, 40*(1), 55S–63S.

Niemi, M.-L., Laaksonen, R., Kotila, M., & Waltimo, O. (1988). Quality of life 4 years after stroke. *Stroke, 19*, 1101–1107.

Nilsson, A., Aniansson, A., & Grimby, G. (2000). Rehabilitation needs and disability in community living stroke survivors two years after stroke. *Topics in Stroke Rehabilitation, 6*(4), 30–47.

Oxenham, D., Sheard, C., & Adams, R. (1995). Comparison of clinician and spouse perceptions of the handicap of aphasia: Everybody understands 'understanding'. *Aphasiology, 9*(5), 477–493.

Parr, S. (1995). Everyday reading and writing in aphasia: Role change and the influence of pre-morbid literacy practice. *Aphasiology, 9*(3), 223–238.

Parr, S., Byng, S., & Gilpin, S., with Ireland, C. (1997). *Talking about aphasia.* Philadelphia: Open University Press.

Pope, A. M., & Tarlov, A. R. (1991). *Disability in America: Towards a national agenda for prevention.* Washington, DC: National Academy Press.

Pound, C., Parr, S., Lindsay, J., & Woolf, C. (2000). *Beyond aphasia: Therapies for living with communication disability.* Bicester, UK: Winslow Press.

Records, N. L., & Baldwin, K. (1996). *A tool to measure "quality of life" of aphasic individuals.* Paper presented at the 1996 ASHA Annual Convention, Pennsylvania.

Reitzes, D. G., Mutran, E. J., & Verrill, L. A. (1995). Activities and self-esteem: Continuing the development of activity theory. *Research on Aging, 17*(3), 260–277.

Resnick, H., Fries, B. E., & Verbrugge, L. M. (1997). Windows to their world: The effect of sensory impairments on social engagement and activity time in nursing home residents. *Journal of Gerontology, 52B*(3), S135–S144.

Robinson-Smith, G., Johnston, M., & Allen, J. (2000). Self-care self-efficacy, quality of life, and depression after stroke. *Archives of Physical Medicine and Rehabilitation, 81*, 460–464.

Rogers, M., Alarcon, N., Olswang, L. (1999). Aphasia management considered in the context of the World Health Organization model of disablements. *Physical Medicine and Rehabilitation Clinics of North America, 10*(4), 907–923.

Ronnberg, L. (1998). Quality of life in nursing home residents: An intervention study of the effect of mental stimulation through an audiovisual programme. *Age and Ageing, 27*(3), 393–397.

Ross, K., & Wertz, R. (2001). Possibly delineating influence on differentiating normal from aphasic performance. *Journal of Communication Disorders, 34*(1–2), 115–130.

Ryff, C., (1989). Happiness is everything, or is it? Explorations on the meaning of well-being. *Journal of Personality and Social Psychology, 57*(6), 1069–1081.

Salomon, G., Vesterager, V., & Jagd, M. (1988). Age-related hearing difficulties: (I) Hearing impairment, disability, and handicap – a controlled study. *Audiology, 27*, 164–178.

Sarno, M. (1997). Quality of life in aphasia in the first post-stroke year. *Aphasiology, 11*(7), 665–679.

Schuling, J., Greidanus, J., & Meyboom-De Jong, B. (1993). Measuring functional status of stroke patients with the Sickness Impact Profile. *Disability and Rehabilitation, 15*(1), 19–23.

Scott, I. U., Smiddy, W. E., Schiffman, J., Feuer, W. J., & Pappas, C. J. (1999). Quality of life of low-vision patients and the impact of low-vision services. *American Journal of Ophthalmology, 128*(1), 54–62.

Sheik, J., & Yesavage, J. (1986). Geriatric Depression Scale (GDS): Recent evidence and development of a shorter version. *Clinical Gerontology, 5*, 165–172.

Stephens, D., & Hetu, R. (1991). Impairment, disability and handicap in audiology: Towards a consensus. *Audiology, 30,* 185–200.

Stephens, D., & Zhao, F. (1996). Hearing impairment: Special needs of the elderly. *Folia Phoniatrica et Logopaedica, 48,* 137–142.

Tate, D. G., Dijkers, M., & Johnson-Greene, L. (1996). Outcome measures in quality of life. *Topics in Stroke Rehabilitation, 2*(4), 1–17.

Thelander, M., Hoen, B., & Worsley, J. (1994). *York-Durham Aphasia Centre: Report on the evaluation of effectiveness of a community program for aphasic adults.* Ontario: York-Durham Aphasia Centre.

Unger, J., McAvay, G., Bruce, M., Berkman, L., & Seeman, T. (1999). Variation in the impact of social network characteristics on physical functioning in elderly persons: MacArthur studies of successful aging. *Journal of Gerontology, 54B*(5), S245–S251.

Wade, D. T., Legh-Smith, J., & Langton Hewer, R. (1985). Social activities after stroke: Measurement and natural history using the Frenchay Activities Index. *International Rehabilitation Medicine, 7,* 176–181.

Ware, J. J., & Sherbourne, C. D. (1992). The MOS 36–item short-form survey (SF-36): I Conceptual framework and item selection. *Medical Care, 30,* 473–483.

Williams, L., Weinberger, M., Harris, L., Clark, D., & Biller, J., (1999). Development of a Stroke-Specific Quality of Life Scale. *Stroke, 30,* 1362–1369.

World Health Organisation. (1997). *WHOQOL: Measuring quality of life.* Geneva: WHO.

World Health Organisation. (1998). *ICIDH-2: International Classification of Impairments, Activities, and Participation: A manual of dimensions of disablement and functioning, beta-1 draft for field trials: An introduction.* Retrieved on January 5, 1998 from the World Wide Web: *http://www.who.ch/programmes/mnh/mnh/ems/icidh/introduction.htm.*

Worrall, L. (1999). *FCTP: Functional Communication Therapy Planner.* Bicester, UK: Winslow.

Wyller, T. B. (1997). Disability models in geriatrics: Comprehensive rather than competing models should be promoted. *Disability and Rehabilitation, 19*(11), 480–483.

Wyller, T., Sveen, U., Sodring, K., Pettersen, A., & Bautz-Holter, E. (1997). Subjective well-being one year after stroke. *Clinical Rehabilitation, 11,* 139–145.

Yoon, H. (1997). Factors affecting quality of life of the Korean aged stroke patients. *International Journal of Aging and Human Development, 44*(3), 167–181.

Zemva, N. (1999). Aphasic patients and their families: Wishes and limits. *Aphasiology, 13*(3), 219–234.

APPENDIX 1

This appendix contains the regression coefficients, probabilities, and variance explained by communication variables in QOL subscales in aphasic participants.

Predictor variables	QOL subscale predicted
Near vision (-3.3, $p = .002$; $r^2 = .41$) with emotional health (-2.6, $p = .02$; $r^2 = .12$)	SF-36 Physical functioning
Social activities (2.8, $p = .01$; $r^2 = .26$) with emotional health (-2.8, $p = .01$; $r^2 = .19$)	SF-36 Role physical
Near vision (-2.2, $p = .04$; $r^2 = .28$) with emotional health (-5.7, $p = .000$; $r^2 = .41$)	SF-36 General health
Social activities (2.1, $p = .05$; $r^2 = .12$) with emotional health (-6.7, $p = .000$; $r^2 = .56$)	SF-36 General health
Near vision (-2.1, $p = .05$; $r^2 = .28$) with emotional health (-4.1, $p = .000$; $r^2 = .29$)	SF-36 Social functioning
CADL-2 (1.9, $p = .07$, $r^2 = .25$) with emotional health (-4.7, $p = .000$; $r^2 = .54$)	SF-36 Social functioning
Near vision ($z = -1.9$) with emotional health ($z = -3$)	COOP Physical fitness
BNT ($z = -3.6$)	COOP Feelings
WAB AQ ($z = -2.8$)	COOP Feelings

Hearing ($z = 2.4$) [reverse relationship]	COOP Feelings
Hearing ($z = -2.7$)	COOP Daily activities
BNT ($z = 2.4$) with emotional health ($z = -4.8$)	COOP Social activities
Near vision ($z = -2.4$) with emotional health ($z = -4.2$)	COOP Social activities
Hearing ($z = -2.1$) with emotional health ($z = -4.7$)	COOP Social activities
WAB AQ ($z = 2.6$) with emotional health ($z = -4.6$)	COOP Social activities
CADL-2 ($z = 3.8$) with emotional health ($z = -4.3$)	COOP Social activities
Social activities ($z = 2.6$)	COOP Social activities
Distance vision ($z = -2.7$)	COOP Change in health
Total social network ($z = 3.3$)	COOP Change in health
Near vision ($z = -2.1$) with emotional health ($z = -3.7$)	COOP Quality of life
CADL-2 ($z = 2.1$) with emotional health ($z = -2.9$)	COOP Quality of life
Emotional health (-3.6, $p = .001$; $r^2 = .48$), near vision (-2.1, $p = .05$; $r^2 = .1$) and age (1.5, $p = .2$, $r^2 = .003$)	Total well-being
Bs near vision corrected for age ($F = 5$, $p = .004$, $r^2 = .47$) [regression coefficient is negative]	Autonomy
Bs near vision ($F = 4$, $p = .02$, $r^2 = .29$) [regression is negative] and bs social network ($F = 5$, $p = .01$, $r^2 = .36$)	Environmental mastery
Bs spontaneous speech ($F = 2.4$, $p = .07$, $r^2 = .29$) and CADL-2 ($F = 2.1$, $p = .11$, $r^2 = .26$)	Personal growth
WAB AQ group 1 (3.4, $p = .002$, $r^2 = .21$); WAB AQ group 2 (3.8, $p = .000$, $r^2 = .41$)	Positive relations with others
Emotional health (-2.4, $p = .03$, $r^2 = .34$), WAB AQ group 1 (3.5, $p = .001$, $r^2 = .05$) and WAB AQ group 2 (3.1, $p = .004$, $r^2 = .3$)	Self-acceptance

Relationships between communication and well-being used some b-spline (bs) curves of the communication variables. As four degrees of freedom was used, four separate regression coefficients were generated. Therefore F values rather than regression coefficients were reported for b-spline variables.

All but two of the above associations were significant at $p < .05$ level. Two associations were retained by the modelling technique even though they did not meet this alpha level.

WAB AQ scores were related to Postive Relations with Others, but exploratory data analysis plots indicated two WAB AQ clusters. Twenty-five cases were classified as group one, and the remaining five as group two. The results reported in the Appendix above account for these two groups. Cluster differences also existed between WAB AQ and Self-acceptance data, wherein group one had 23 cases and group two had 7 cases.

APHASIOLOGY, 2003, *17* (4), 355–364

Quality of life with and without aphasia

Katherine B. Ross

*Carl T. Hayden Veterans Affairs Medical Center, Arizona, and
Arizona State University, USA*

Robert T. Wertz

*Department of Veterans Affairs Tennessee Valley Healthcare System, and
Vanderbilt University School of Medicine, USA*

Background: Although the social approach to managing aphasia is designed to improve the quality of life (QOL) of the aphasic person, the influence of being aphasic on different facets of QOL is unknown.

Aims: To delineate socially valid therapy targets, we examined 24 facets of QOL proposed by the World Health Organisation (WHO) to determine which facets differentiate QOL between aphasic and nonaphasic people.

Methods & Procedures: A prospective, observational, non-randomised group design was employed. Two measures—the WHO QOL Instrument, Short Form (WHOQOL-BREF) and the Psychosocial Well-Being Index (PWI)—were administered to 18 adults with chronic aphasia and 18 nonaphasic adults. Indices of determination (ID) and degrees of overlap (DO) were calculated to determine which of the 24 facets were best in differentiating between the aphasic and nonaphasic groups.

Outcomes & Results: Facets within three domains—level of independence, social relationships, and environment—were best in distinguishing QOL between the aphasic and nonaphasic groups.

Conclusion: Therapy that focuses on situation-specific communication and societal participation appears to be most appropriate for enhancing the QOL of people with chronic aphasia.

The anticipated outcome of a social approach to aphasia management is improved quality of life (Simmons-Mackie, 2000). Quality of life (QOL) is defined as individuals' "perceptions of their position in life in the context of the culture and value systems where they live and in relation to their goals, expectations, standards and concerns" (The WHOQOL Group, 1996, p. 354) and is presumed to be inherently influenced by disability, physical health, psychological state, level of independence, social relationships, environmental factors, and personal beliefs (De Haan, Horn, Limburg, Van Der Meulen, & Bossuyt, 1993; The WHOQOL Group, 1996). Aphasic stroke survivors report sig-

Address correspondence to: Katherine B. Ross, Carl T. Hayden Veterans Affairs Medical Center, Audiology and Speech Pathology Department (CS/126), 650 E. Indian School Road, Phoenix, AZ 85012-1892, USA. Email: katherine.ross3@med.va.gov

This study was conducted at the Veterans Affairs Medical Center, Nashville, Tennessee and was supported in part by a pre-doctoral fellowship from the Department of Veterans Affairs and by the Vanderbilt University School of Medicine Department of Hearing and Speech Sciences. We thank Daniel Ashmead, PhD, Fred Bess, PhD, Patrick J. Doyle, PhD, Frank Freemon, MD, PhD, and Ralph Ohde, PhD for valuable discussion.

http://www.tandf.co.uk/journals/pp/02687038.html

DOI:10.1080/02687030244000716

nificantly lower overall QOL than do non-brain-injured (NBI) adults (Ross & Wertz, 2000). However, the difference in various facets of QOL between aphasic and nonaphasic people has not been determined. Consequently, evidence-based treatment targets for improving the QOL of aphasic people are not known.

Much of the aphasia QOL literature has reported specific, psychosocial consequences of aphasia rather than systematic, prospective examinations of variables conceptualised to predict QOL (Herrmann & Wallesch, 1989). For example, reports obtained from patients, spouses, and clinicians suggest that loss of independence (Herrmann & Wallesch, 1990); inability to work (Herrmann & Wallesch, 1989); loss of self-identity (Brumfitt, 1993); and social isolation (Artes & Hoops, 1976; Herrmann & Wallesch, 1989; Kinsella & Duffy, 1978; Sarno, 1993) are devastating effects of chronic aphasia. However, specific psychosocial symptoms experienced by aphasic adults may or may not differ from those of their normally-ageing peers. Comprehensive comparisons between aphasic and non-aphasic people have not been reported. Thus, the appropriateness of different facets of QOL as therapy targets is undetermined.

The influence of being aphasic on different facets of QOL is also uncertain. Relevant stakeholders (e.g., patients, caregivers, and healthcare providers) disagree as to the burden associated with different facets and their importance as therapeutic objectives. Sneeuw, Aaronson, de Haan, and Limburg (1997) compared quality of life data obtained from stroke survivors and their significant others, using the Sickness Impact Profile (SIP) (Bergner, Bobbitt, Carter, & Gilson, 1981). Proxies systematically rated stroke survivors as having more QOL impairments than did stroke survivors themselves. Hermann and Wallesch (1990) asked 22 rehabilitation experts from various professions (e.g., occupational therapy, speech pathology, neurology) to rank 10 psychosocial facets that compose the Code-Müller Protocols (CMP) (Code & Müller, 1992) according to relevance in aphasia rehabilitation. The obtained rankings appeared to be influenced by the therapy goals and requirements of the various professions. Physiotherapists, for example, placed much greater emphasis than other experts on patients achieving "independence of others". Hemsley and Code (1996) administered the CMP to chronically aphasic patients, their spouses, and their speech pathologists. Prioritisation of emotional and psychosocial factors differed considerably among individuals. By definition, assessment of quality of life requires an individual's subjective evaluation of his or her life situation (Brown & Gordon, 1999). Socially valid treatment planning requires a client's selection of intervention targets (Simmons-Mackie, 2000). Thus, the relative impact of different facets on an aphasic individual's QOL must be determined by the aphasic person.

To measure quality of life in patient populations, a combination of generic and disease-specific measures is recommended (Hirsch & Holland, 2000; McSweeney, 1990; Spilker, 1996). The World Health Organisation's Quality of Life Instrument (WHOQOL-100), a generic measure, was developed to represent a "reliable, valid, and responsive assessment of quality of life that is applicable across cultures" (The WHOQOL Group, 1998a, p. 1569). It includes 24 facets (four questions each) universally regarded by 15 field centres around the world as important in assessing QOL, as well as four general questions that address general QOL and health. Facets are grouped into six domains—Physical, Psychological, Independence, Social, Environment, and Spiritual. A shorter version, the WHOQOL-BREF, contains 26 items grouped into four domains and is presently available as a field trial version (The WHOQOL Group, 1998b). The Psychosocial Well-being Index (PWI) (Lyon et al., 1997), a disease-specific measure, is a non-standardised, 11-item questionnaire developed to assess key constructs of QOL with aphasia. Generic measures permit comparison of QOL data between groups, whereas disease-specific scales are sensitive to problems relevant to specific populations (Hirsch & Holland, 2000; McSweeney, 1990; Spilker, 1996).

The purpose of this investigation was to determine differences between aphasic and nonaphasic people on different facets of QOL to support selection of socially valid therapy targets for aphasic people. We used a combination of generic and disease-specific measures to examine 24 facets of QOL, proposed by the World Health Organisation Quality of Life Group (1996), in individuals with chronic aphasia and non-brain-injured controls. The primary research question was, Which facets best differentiate QOL between people with and without aphasia?

METHOD

Participants

Study participants met the following selection criteria. All were between 40 and 80 years of age and were premorbidly literate in English. All participants had: (1) hearing no worse than an estimated 40 decibel (dB) speech recognition threshold (SRT) in the better ear as determined by the Carhart method (i.e., the average of pure tone thresholds at 500 and 1000 Hz, minus 2 dB, Carhart, 1971); (2) corrected visual acuity no worse than 20/ 100 in the better eye as determined by a pocket-sized Snellen chart; (3) one upper extremity sufficiently intact to point, gesture, and write; and, (4) no coexisting medical or psychological disorders that would interfere with participation in the study, including no active treatment for substance abuse.

Participants with aphasia had: (1) a history of one or more strokes, with the most recent stroke occurring at least 6 months prior to entry in the study; (2) brain damage confined to the left hemisphere; (3) no history of other disease that would affect communicative ability; and (4) a diagnosis of aphasia, based on the following operational definition (Rosenbek, LaPointe, & Wertz, 1989, p. 53):

> Aphasia is an impairment, due to acquired ... damage of the central nervous system, of the ability to comprehend and formulate language. It is a multimodality disorder represented by a variety of impairments in auditory comprehension, reading, oral-expressive language, and writing. The disrupted language may be influenced by physiological inefficiency or impaired recognition, but it cannot be explained by dementia, sensory loss, or motor dysfunction.

Diagnoses of aphasia were determined by the principal investigators, certified speech-language pathologists with extensive experience in the diagnosis and treatment of individuals with aphasia. The individuals with aphasia in this study were at least 6 months post-stroke.

Non-brain-injured (NBI) controls had no history of brain injury or other disease that would affect communicative ability. Absence of brain damage in NBI controls was based on self-reported medical history, whereas presence of brain damage in participants with aphasia was verified by radiologists' interpretation of computed tomography (CT) and/or magnetic resonance imaging (MRI) scans.

Table 1 shows participants' demographic information. Thirteen males (72%) and five females (28%) composed each group. Age and educational level did not differ significantly ($p < .05$) between groups. Twelve (67%) of the participants with aphasia had suffered ischaemic strokes, four (22%) had suffered haemorrhagic strokes, and two (11%) had suffered ruptured aneurysms. Administration of the WAB Aphasia Quotient (AQ) classifies all individuals scoring below an arbitrary cutoff of 93.8 as having one of eight

TABLE 1
Demographic data for non-brain-injured (NBI) (n = 18) and chronically aphasic
(n = 18) participants

Variable	Mean	Range	SD
Age (years)			
NBI participants	60.61	41–75	9.42
Aphasic participants	60.78	48–79	7.84
Educational level (years)			
NBI participants	15.06	7–22	3.52
Aphasic participants	13.58	8–18	2.80
Severity of impairment (WAB AQ[a])			
NBI participants	99.02	95.20–100.00	1.40
Aphasic participants	72.62	13.60–99.00	26.48
Time post-stroke (months)			
Aphasic participants	42.78	6–144	40.44

[a] Western Aphasia Battery Aphasia Quotient (range, 0–100, Kertesz, 1982)

types of aphasia. In the current sample of participants with aphasia, five (28%) were classified as having anomic aphasia, four (22%) as having conduction aphasia, four (22%) as "not aphasic", three (17%) as having Broca's aphasia, and two (11%) as having Wernicke's aphasia. The four individuals classified as "not aphasic" exhibited persistent, mild impairment in verbal expression and auditory comprehension and more significant impairment in reading and/or writing. The WAB, however, uses only two of four language modalities, auditory comprehension and verbal expression, to diagnose and classify aphasia. The WAB performance of all (100%) NBI controls classified them as "not aphasic".

Design and procedure

A prospective, observational, non-randomised group design was employed. All participants were administered two QOL measures—the WHOQOL-BREF and the PWI. Quality of life data were collected using a written questionnaire format. If an individual was unable to complete a questionnaire independently, an interviewer-assisted format was employed. If necessary, repetition, rephrasing, and item-specific examples were used to enhance the validity of aphasic responses. Thus, each participant provided his or her own personal assessment of QOL.

Statistical analyses

To determine which facets best distinguish QOL with and without aphasia, an index of determination (ID) and degree of overlap (DO) were calculated for each item. The index of determination (Young, 1976) uses regression analysis concepts to measure the degree to which being classified, a priori, as "aphasic" or "normal" predicts performance on a given measure. The degree of overlap represents the percentage of aphasic participants scoring at or above the minimum expected score for 95% of NBI controls. Duffy and Keith (1980) suggest that a large index of determination or a small percentage of overlap is associated with good discriminatory power in distinguishing "aphasic" from "normal" performance.

TABLE 2
Overall QOL in non-brain-injured (NBI) (n = 18) and chronically aphasic (n = 18) participants

Measure	Mean	Range	SD	Mean difference	95% C. I.[a] of difference	t(34)
WHOQOL-BREF Transformed total						
NBI participants	108.44	94.00–125.00	10.02			
Aphasic participants	96.11	68.00–124.00	14.05	12.23	4.07–20.60	3.03**
WHOQOL-BREF overall QOL and						
general health rating						
NBI participants	8.44	6.00–10.00	1.58			
Aphasic participants	7.22	4.00–10.00	1.52	1.22	0.17–2.27	2.37*
PWI total						
NBI participants	36.33	28.00–42.00	3.40			
Aphasic participants	31.72	22.00–41.00	5.90	4.61	1.35–2.87	2.87**

[a] Confidence interval.
*$p < .05$ **$p < .01$

RESULTS

Table 2 shows group comparisons on the QOL measures. The chronically aphasic group reported significantly lower overall QOL on the WHOQOL-BREF transformed total score ($p < .01$), WHOQOL-BREF Overall QOL and General Health Rating ($p < .05$), and the PWI total score ($p < .01$), than did NBI controls.

Table 3 shows the discriminative ability of each QOL facet. To determine which facets best differentiate QOL with and without aphasia, individual facets of QOL may be ranked according to obtained indices of determination and degrees of overlap. Six facets fell within the top 25th percentile for both indicators (i.e., largest index of determination and smallest degree of overlap) and thus best differentiate QOL with and without aphasia. The best determinant was activities of daily living (ID, 14–33%; DO, 45–89%), followed by opportunities for acquiring new information and skills (ID, 24%; DO, 45%), social support (ID, 31%; DO, 67%), mobility (ID, 19–29%; DO, 67–83%), work capacity (ID, 23%; DO, 78%), and sexual activity (ID, 17%; DO, 78%).

Six facets fell within the top 50th percentile for both indicators and thus discriminated QOL with and without aphasia less powerfully: self-esteem (ID, 1–22%; DO, 89–100%), followed by health and social care accessibility and quality (ID, 20%; DO, 89%), transport (ID, 15%; DO, 78%), spirituality/religion/personal beliefs (ID, 2–14%; DO, 72–89%), positive feelings (ID, 2–6%; DO, 89%), and personal relationships (ID, 0–10%; DO, 83–100%).

Other facets demonstrated negligible discriminatory power in distinguishing "aphasic" from "normal" QOL: dependence on medicinal substances and medical aids (ID, 9%; DO, 94%), followed by thinking/learning/memory/concentration (ID, 15%; DO, 100%), energy and fatigue (ID, 2%; DO, 83%), bodily image and appearance (ID, 1%; DO, 89%), home environment (ID, 4%; DO, 94%), freedom/physical safety/security (ID, 3%; DO, 94%), financial resources (ID, 3%; DO, 100%), sleep and rest (ID, 0%; DO, 94%), negative feelings (ID, 0%; DO, 94%), pain and discomfort (ID, 0%; DO, 100%), participation in and opportunities for recreation/leisure activity (ID, 0%; DO, 100%), and physical environment (ID, 0%; DO, 100%).

TABLE 3
Facets of QOL in non-brain-injured (NBI) (n=18) and chronically aphasic (n=18) participants

QOL facet	Index of determination (%)	Degree of overlap (%)
Physical domain		
Pain and discomfort		
WHOQOL-BREF Item 3	0	100
Energy and fatigue		
WHOQOL-BREF Item 10	2	83
Sleep and rest		
WHOQOL-BREF Item 16	0	94
Psychological domain		
Positive feelings		
WHOQOL-BREF Item 5	2	89
PWI Item 2	6	89
Thinking, learning, memory, and concentration		
WHOQOL-BREF Item 7	15	100
Self-esteem		
WHOQOL-BREF Item 19	22	89
PWI Item 7	5	100
PWI Item 9	1	100
Bodily image and appearance		
WHOQOL-BREF Item 11	1	89
Negative feelings		
WHOQOL-BREF Item 26	0	94
Level of independence domain		
Mobility		
WHOQOL-BREF Item 15	29	83
PWI Item 6	19	67
Activities of daily living		
WHOQOL-BREF Item 17	33	45
PWI Item 4	7	67
PWI Item 5	14	89
Dependence on medicinal substances and medical aids		
WHOQOL-BREF Item 4	9	94
Work capacity		
WHOQOL-BREF Item 18	23	78
Social relationships domain		
Personal relationships		
WHOQOL-BREF Item 20	10	89
PWI Item 8	0	100
PWI Item 10	3	83
PWI Item 11	10	100
Social support		
WHOQOL-BREF Item 22	31	67
Sexual activity		
WHOQOL-BREF Item 21	17	78
Environment domain		
Freedom, physical safety, and security		
WHOQOL-BREF Item 8	3	94
Home environment		
WHOQOL-BREF Item 23	4	94
Financial resources		
WHOQOL-BREF Item 12	3	100
Health and social care: Accessibility and quality		
WHOQOL-BREF Item 24	20	89

Continued opposite

TABLE 3 *(continued)*

QOL facet	Index of determination (%)	Degree of overlap (%)
Opportunities for acquiring new information and skills		
WHOQOL-BREF Item 13	24	45
Participation in and opportunities for recreation/leisure activity		
WHOQOL-BREF Item 14	0	100
PWI Item 3	0	100
Physical environment		
WHOQOL-BREF Item 9	0	100
Transport		
WHOQOL-BREF Item 25	15	78
Spiritual domain		
Spirituality/religion/personal beliefs		
WHOQOL-BREF Item 6	2	72
PWI Item 1	14	89

Seven facets were assessed by both QOL measures. For four facets, the WHOQOL-BREF and PWI were comparably sensitive to differences between groups: positive feelings (WHOQOL-BREF ID/DO, 2%/89%; PWI ID/DO, 6%/89%); mobility (WHOQOL-BREF ID/DO, 29%/83%; PWI ID/DO, 19%/67%); personal relationships (WHOQOL-BREF ID/DO, 10%/89%; PWI ID/DO, 0–10%/83 100%); and, leisure opportunities (both ID/DO, 0%/100%). For two facets, the WHOQOL-BREF was most sensitive: self-esteem (WHOQOL-BREF ID/DO, 22%/89%; PWI ID/DO, 1–5%/100%); activities of daily living (WHOQOL-BREF ID/DO, 33%/45%; PWI ID/DO, 7–14%/67–89%). For one facet, the PWI was most sensitive to differences in QOL with and without aphasia: spirituality/religion/personal beliefs (WHOQOL-BREF ID/DO, 2%/72%; PWI ID/DO, 14%/89%).

DISCUSSION

The purpose of this study was to determine which of 24 facets proposed by the World Health Organisation Quality of Life Group (1996) best differentiate QOL with and without aphasia. Various facets of QOL may be grouped into six domains: physical, psychological, level of independence, social relationships, and environment (The WHOQOL Group, 1996). Data indicate that facets within three domains—level of independence, social relationships, and environment—best distinguish QOL between the aphasic and nonaphasic groups. Within the domain of level of independence, respondents' ability to perform daily activities, to get around, and to work, best differentiates between normal and aphasic QOL. Within the domain of social relationships, respondents' satisfaction with support received from friends and with their sex lives, best distinguishes QOL between the groups. Within the environmental domain, accessibility—of information, health services, and transportation—best discriminates between QOL with and without aphasia. Our results concur with previous reports that loss of independence (Hermann & Wallesch, 1990); inability to work (Herrmann & Wallesch, 1989); and social isolation (Artes & Hoops, 1976; Herrmann & Wallesch, 1989; Kinsella & Duffy, 1978; Sarno, 1993) are psychosocial burdens of chronic aphasia.

The development of aphasia therapy has traditionally been guided by the medical model of disability, which focuses on functional limitations of the patient. In this model, the goal of therapy is to decrease the individual's impairment(s) and restore maximum language function (e.g., Pound, Parr, Linsday, & Woolf, 2001). However, data indicate that the experience of living with chronic aphasia may be most affected by facets other than severity of language-based disability. Ross and Wertz (2002) found no significant relationships between severity of language-based disability (as measured by the Porch Index of Communicative Ability, PICA, Porch, 1967; WAB; Communication Activities of Daily Living – Second Edition, CADL-2, Holland, Frattali, & Fromm, 1999; and the American Speech-Language-Hearing Association Functional Assessment of Communication Skills for Adults, ASHA FACS, Frattali, Thompson, Holland, Wohl, & Ferketic, 1995) and QOL with mild to moderate aphasia (as measured by the WHOQOL-BREF and PWI). Hemsley and Code (1996) administered the CMP to five individuals with mild to moderate aphasia at 3 and 9 months post-onset. Ten factors considered relevant to psychosocial adjustment to aphasia were ranked and weighted by each respondent. While all participants initially attributed high importance to speech therapy, only two patients still considered it to be a priority at 9 months post-stroke. Our data concur. In our sample, the QOL facet most related to traditional speech-language therapy targets—"thinking, learning, memory, and concentration"—discriminated poorly between quality of life with and without chronic aphasia. Facets related to social relationships and environmental barriers, however, were among the best predictors of group membership.

Thus, a growing body of evidence suggests that the social model of disability might more appropriately guide the development of speech-language therapy for later stages of recovery. In this model, disability stems from the failure of the social and physical environment to account for the needs of individuals with aphasia, rather than from the functional limitations of patients themselves (Abberly, 1991; Finkelstein & French, 1993; Pound et al., 2001). Simmons-Mackie (2000) and Byng, Pound, and Parr (2000) have incorporated the social model of disability in the development of interrelated goals of therapy. Objectives include enhancing communication; identifying and dismantling barriers to social participation; maximising a healthy psychological state; encouraging autonomy and choice; and promoting advocacy and social action. Although the needs of individuals with aphasia may vary at any point in time, our data suggest that chronically aphasic individuals might benefit especially from continued language therapy to enhance communication for specific situations (e.g., to facilitate access to public transportation systems) and from efforts to expand and enrich participation in society (e.g., by weakening barriers to and enhancing personal identity within relationships).

Unresolved issues in the current measurement of QOL prohibit more specific recommendations. First, no comprehensive, conceptually coherent, psychometrically sound assessment of QOL with aphasia exists. Measures designed *de novo* to test single hypotheses may not measure all QOL domains important to aphasic people (Spitzer, 1987; Veldhuyzen Van Zanten, 1991). We observed that the PWI, which was developed to measure the outcome of a communication partners therapy, was less sensitive than the WHOQOL-BREF in differentiating QOL with and without aphasia. Second, although the WHOQOL-BREF does assess six domains of QOL, respondents are not asked to rank or weight the significance of items. Thus, the relative importance of each QOL domain to an individual cannot be determined. Third, even comprehensive instruments may omit certain constructs that are important to individual patients' QOL (Gill & Feinstein, 1994). Respondents should be provided with an opportunity to supplement standardised items with those regarded as personally relevant. Fourth, our data were collected from a relatively small and homogeneous group of adults with mild to moderately severe chronic aphasia. To permit therapy suggestions specific to time post-onset of recovery, aphasic profile (type and severity), and personal factors (e.g., coping style, dispositional optimism), further study, using larger sample sizes and causal modelling techniques (Duffy, 1993), is essential.

Finally, a social model of aphasia management does not advocate abandonment of impairment-based assessment or language therapy. Rather, practitioners advocate expansion of traditional practices to incorporate the achievement of individuals' social and communication goals (Simmons-Mackie, 2000). By promoting linguistic, psychological, and social recovery as defined and prioritised by each client (Pound et al., 2001), speech-language pathologists might best enhance quality of life with aphasia.

REFERENCES

Abberly, P. (1991). The significance of the OPCS disability surveys. In M. Oliver (Ed.), *Social work: Disabled people and disabling environments*. London: Jessica Kingsley.

Artes, R., & Hoops, R. (1976). Problems of aphasic and nonaphasic stroke patients as identified and evaluated by patients' wives. In Y. Lebrun & R. Hoops (Eds.), *Recovery in aphasics* (pp. 31–45). Amsterdam: Swets & Zeitlinger.

Bergner, M., Bobbitt, R. A., Carter, W. B., & Gilson, B. S. (1981). The Sickness Impact Profile: Development and final revision of a health status measure. *Medical Care, 19*, 787–805.

Brown, M., & Gordon, W. A. (1999). Quality of life as a construct in health and disability research. *The Mount Sinai Journal of Medicine, 66*, 160–169.

Brumfitt, S. (1993). Losing your sense of self: What aphasia can do. *Aphasiology, 7*, 569–591.

Byng, S., Pound, C., & Parr, S. (2000). Living with aphasia: A framework for therapy interventions. In I. Papathanasiou (Ed.), *Acquired neurogenic communication disorders: A clinical perspective* (pp. 49–75). London: Whurr Publishers.

Carhart, R. (1971). Observations on relations between thresholds for pure tones and speech. *Journal of Speech and Hearing Disorders, 36*, 476–483.

Code, C., & Müller, D. J. (1992). *The Code-Müller Protocols: Assessing perceptions of psychosocial adjustment to aphasia and related disorders*. London: Whurr Publishers.

De Haan, R., Horn, J., Limburg, M., Van Der Meulen, J., & Bossuyt, P. (1993). A comparison of five stroke scales with measures of disability, handicap, and quality of life. *Stroke, 24*, 1178–1181.

Duffy, J. (1993). Path analysis. In M. L. Lemme (Ed.), *Clinical aphasiology, 21* (pp. 47–57). Austin, TX: Pro-Ed.

Duffy, J. R., & Keith, R. C. (1980). Performance of non-brain injured adults on the PICA: Descriptive data and a comparison to patients with aphasia. *Aphasia-Apraxia-Agnosia, 2*, 1–30.

Finkelstein, V., & French, S. (1993). Towards a psychology of disability. In J. Swain, V. Finkelstein, S. French, & M. Oliver (Eds.), *Disabling barriers—enabling environments*. London: Sage.

Frattali, C., Thompson, C. K., Holland, A. L., Wohl, C. B., & Ferketic, M. K. (1995). *American Speech-Language-Hearing Association assessment of functional communication skills for adults*. Rockville, MD: American Speech-Language-Hearing Association.

Gill, T. M., & Feinstein, A. R. (1994). A critical appraisal of the quality of quality-of-life measurements. *Journal of the American Medical Association, 272*, 619–626.

Hemsley, G., & Code, C. (1996). Interactions between recovery in aphasia, emotional and psychosocial factors in subjects with aphasia, their significant others, and speech pathologists. *Disability and Rehabilitation, 18*, 567–584.

Herrmann, M., & Wallesch, C.-W. (1989). Psychosocial changes and psychosocial adjustment with chronic and severe non-fluent aphasia. *Aphasiology, 3*, 513–526.

Herrmann, M., & Wallesch, C.-W. (1990). Expectations of psychosocial adjustment in aphasia: A MAUT study with the Code-Müller Scale of Psychosocial Adjustment. *Aphasiology, 4*, 527–538.

Hirsch, F. M., & Holland, A. L. (2000). Beyond activity: Measuring participation in society and quality of life. In L. E. Worrall & C. M. Frattali (Eds.), *Neurogenic communication disorders: A functional approach* (pp. 35–54). New York: Thieme Publishers.

Holland, A. L., Frattali, C., & Fromm, D. (1999). *Communication activities of daily living—Second Edition*. Austin: Pro-ed.

Kertesz, A. (1982). *Western aphasia battery*. New York: Grune & Stratton.

Kinsella, G., & Duffy, F. D. (1978). The spouse of the aphasic patient. In Y. Lebrun & R. Hoops (Eds.), *The management of aphasia* (pp. 26–49). Amsterdam: Swets & Zeitlinger.

Lyon, J. G., Cariski, D., Keisler, L., Rosenbek, J., Levine, R., Kumpula, J., Ryff, C., Coyne, S., & Blanc, M. (1997). Communication partners: Enhancing participation in life and communication for adults with aphasia in natural settings. *Aphasiology*, *11*, 693–708.

McSweeney, A. J. (1990). Quality-of-life assessment in neuropsychology. In D. E. Tupper & K. D. Cicerone (Eds.), *The neuropsychology of everyday life: Assessment and basic competencies* (pp. 185–217). Boston: Kluwer Academic Publishers.

Porch, B. E. (1967). *Porch index of communicative ability*. Palo Alto, CA: Consulting Psychologists Press.

Pound, C., Parr, S., Linsday, J., & Woolf, C. (2001). *Beyond aphasia: Therapies for living with communication disability* (pp. 1–32). Bicester, UK: Speechmark.

Rosenbek, J. C., LaPointe, L. L., & Wertz, R. T. (1989). *Aphasia: A clinical approach*. Boston: College Hill Press.

Ross, K. B., & Wertz, R. T. (2000, November). *Validity of current measures for differentiating normal from aphasic performance*. Poster session presented at the American Speech-Language-Hearing Association Convention, Washington, DC.

Ross, K. B., & Wertz, R. T. (2002). Relationships between language-based disability and quality of life in chronically aphasic adults. *Aphasiology*, *16*, 791–800.

Sarno, M. T. (1993). Aphasia rehabilitation: Psychosocial and ethical considerations. *Aphasiology*, *7*, 321–334.

Simmons-Mackie, N. N. (2000). Social approaches to the management of aphasia. In L. E. Worrall & C. M. Frattali (Eds.), *Neurogenic communication disorders: A functional approach* (pp. 162–185). New York: Thieme Publishers.

Sneeuw, K. C., Aaronson, N. K., de Haan, R. J., & Limburg, M. (1997). Assessing quality of life after stroke: The value and limitations of proxy ratings. *Stroke*, *28*, 1541–1549.

Spilker, B. (1996). Introduction. In B. Spilker (Ed.), *Quality of life and pharmacoeconomics in clinical trials* (2nd ed., pp. 1–10). Philadelphia: Lippincott-Raven.

Spitzer, W. O. (1987). State of science 1986: Quality of life and functional status as target variables for research. *Journal of Chronic Diseases*, *40*, 465–471.

The WHOQOL Group (1996). What quality of life? *World Health Forum*, *17*, 354–356.

The WHOQOL Group. (1998a). The World Health Organization Quality of Life Assessment (WHOQOL): Development and general psychometric properties. *Social Science Medicine*, *46*, 1569–1585.

The WHOQOL Group. (1998b). Development of the World Health Organization WHOQOL-BREF Quality of Life Assessment. *Psychological Medicine*, *28*, 551–558.

Veldhuyzen Van Zanten, S. J. O. (1991). Quality of life as outcome measures in randomized clinical trials: An overview of three general medical journals. *Controlled Clinical Trials*, *12*, 234S–242S.

Young, M. (1976). Application of regression analysis concepts to retrospective research in speech pathology. *Journal of Speech and Hearing Research*, *19*, 5–18.

APHASIOLOGY, 2003, *17* (4), 365–381

Predictors of health-related quality of life (HRQL) in people with chronic aphasia

Katerina Hilari, Richard D. Wiggins, and Penny Roy

City University, London, UK

Sally Byng

Connect – the communication disability network, London, UK

Sarah C. Smith

London School of Hygiene and Tropical Medicine, London, UK

Background: In recent years, quality of life measures have been used increasingly to evaluate the effectiveness of services or interventions. For people with chronic disabilities, research has focused on identifying the main predictors of their health-related quality of life (HRQL), in order to address the issue of how to meet their needs in rehabilitation in a more holistic way.

Aims: This study assessed the main predictors of HRQL in people with chronic aphasia following stroke. We investigated the relationship between HRQL and various demographic and stroke-related variables and other variables that have been associated with HRQL in stroke survivors (e.g., emotional distress, daily activities, social support).

Methods: A cross-sectional design was adopted. A cluster sampling framework was used to recruit participants with chronic aphasia (> 1 year) from three different sites. Questionnaires and assessments on the different variables were administered to all participants by a speech and language therapist, in an interview format. Multiple regression analysis was used to assess what were the main predictors of HRQL in people with aphasia.

Results: Of 95 participants, 83 (87%) were able to self-report on all the assessments. Emotional distress, involvement in home and outdoors activities, extent of communication disability, and number of comorbid conditions explained 52% of the variance in HRQL (adjusted R^2 = .52). Stroke type (infarct vs haemorrhage), time post-onset, and demographic variables (gender, ethnicity, marital status, employment status, and socioeconomic status) were not significantly associated with HRQL in these participants.

Conclusions: Increased distress, reduced involvement in activities, increased communication disability, and comorbidity predict poorer HRQL in people with chronic aphasia after stroke. Service providers need to take these factors into account when designing intervention programmes.

Address correspondence to: Dr Katerina Hilari, Department of Language and Communication Science, City University, Northampton Square, London EC1V 0HB, UK.
Email: K.Hilari@city.ac.uk

This study was funded by the Stroke Association, London, and the Dunhill Medical Trust, London. We are grateful to the SLTs in the recruiting sites for their help and to all the respondents and their families for participating in this study. We would also like to thank Dr Jane Marshall for her helpful comments in reviewing an earlier version of this paper.

http://www.tandf.co.uk/journals/pp/02687038.html   DOI:10.1080/02687030244000725

INTRODUCTION

Evaluating healthcare provision: Patient-based outcomes

In recent decades there has been a paradigm shift in the way health and healthcare provision are conceptualised and evaluated. In 1948, the WHO indicated that health is no longer merely the absence of disease, but rather "a state of complete physical, mental and social well-being". This is a broad conceptualisation and although there is no consensus on an exact definition of health it is generally accepted that it incorporates physical, mental, and social components (Berzon, Hays, & Shumaker, 1993).

This broader conceptualisation of health is reflected in the way healthcare interventions are evaluated. Evaluation has moved beyond the measurement of traditional clinical outcomes such as morbidity and mortality to establishing the effectiveness of interventions based on critical and rigorous scientific evidence using a wide range of outcome measures (NHS Executive, 1996). Another change in recent years is that patients have become increasingly involved in treatment decisions (NHS Executive, 1999) and there is general consensus that patients and carers are "experts" in their own conditions. Patient-based measures of outcome are, therefore, increasingly used in the evaluation of healthcare interventions.

Health-related quality of life (HRQL) and chronic disability

HRQL measures represent one form of patient-based measures. HRQL reflects the impact of a health state on a person's ability to lead a fulfilling life (Bullinger, Anderson, Cella, & Aaronson, 1993). It incorporates the individual's perception of and satisfaction with his/her physical, mental/emotional, family, and social functioning (Berzon et al., 1993; de Haan, Horn, Limburg, Van Der Meulen, & Bossuyt, 1993; Hays, Anderson, & Revicki, 1993).

HRQL measures are particularly useful in the evaluation of healthcare interventions for people with chronic diseases and disabilities. Rehabilitation of people with chronic disabilities has traditionally focused on compensatory programmes (Frey, 1984) but in recent years it has begun to concentrate more on facilitating adaptation to disability and social and community integration (Royal College of Physicians, 2000; Turner, 1990; Wood-Dauphinee & Williams, 1987). Patient-based HRQL measures are particularly suited for the evaluation of healthcare provision in people with chronic disabilities as they allow us to better understand and measure the impact of disease on the patient's life as a whole (Patrick & Erickson, 1993). They also allow us to incorporate the patient's perspective in clinical decision making (Mayou & Bryant, 1993; Wenger, Mattson, Furberg, & Elison, 1984).

Stroke and aphasia

Stroke is the most common cause of long-term adult disability in the world. A number of studies have looked at patient outcomes and quality of life[1] following stroke. In most of

---

[1] Quality of life is a related but broader term than HRQL, often related to a person's culture and value systems (World Health Organisation QOL Assessment Group, 1993) and incorporating factors like a safe environment and material well-being. The healthcare system and its providers usually do not assume responsibility for these more global human concerns although they may be adversely affected by disease (Patrick & Erickson, 1993). Most of the literature reviewed here has actually assessed what is commonly viewed now as HRQL, but has used the term quality of life. In reporting other people's work we have used the terms they used.

these studies quality of life is affected by *depression* (Ahlsio, Britton, & Murray, 1984; Clarke, Black, Badley, Lawrence, & Williams, 1999; Duncan et al., 1997; Jonkman, deWeerd, & Vrijens, 1998; King, 1996; Lofgren, Gustafson, & Nyberg, 1999; Neau et al., 1998; Niemi, Laaksonen, Kotila, & Waltimo, 1988); and *physical disabilities/reduced activities* (Ahlsio et al., 1984; Angeleri, Angeleri, Foschi, Giaquinto, & Nolfe, 1993; Astrom, Adolfsson, Asplund, & Astrom, 1992a; Astrom, Asplund, & Astrom, 1992b; Clarke et al., 1999; Duncan et al., 1997; Ebrahim, Barer, & Nouri, 1986; Jonkman et al., 1998; King, 1996; Kwa, Limburg, & de Haan, 1996; Lofgren et al., 1999; Neau et al., 1998; Niemi et al., 1988; Viitanen, Fugl-Meyer, Bernspaang, & Fugl-Meyer, 1988; Wilkinson et al., 1997).

Other predictors of poor quality of life have included *reduced social support* (Astrom et al., 1992a; Astrom et al., 1992b; King, 1996; Osberg et al., 1988; Viitanen et al., 1988; Wyller, Holmen, Laake, & Laake, 1998); and *cognitive decline* in some studies (Clarke et al., 1999; Jonkman et al., 1998; Niemi et al., 1988) but not in others (Kwa et al., 1996). Out of 14 studies reviewed that included people with aphasia, only two found *aphasia* to be significantly associated with poorer quality of life (Neau et al., 1998, in univariate but not multivariate analysis; Kwa et al., 1996).

Other factors that have been associated with poorer quality of life after stroke are *older age* in some studies (Astrom et al., 1992a; Astrom et al., 1992b; de Haan, Limburg, Van der Meulen, Jacobs, & Aaronson, 1995) but not in others (Ahlsio et al., 1984; Ebrahim et al., 1986; Wyller et al., 1998); increased *comorbidity* (Clarke et al., 1999; de Haan et al., 1995; Duncan et al., 1997); lower *socioeconomic or educational/professional status* (King et al., 1996; Neau et al., 1998); and some *stroke related variables*—e.g., ischaemic and hemispheric stroke in Niemi et al. (1988); supratentorial strokes in de Haan et al. (1995); and larger infarct volume in Kwa et al. (1996).

It is not easy, however, to draw meaningful conclusions from this literature due to a number of methodological and conceptual challenges. In particular, a key methodological challenge in the area of stroke HRQL is that people with aphasia may have difficulty completing self-report assessments. As a result, in some of the studies, people with aphasia were excluded (e.g., Clarke et al., 1999; Duncan et al., 1997; Jonkman et al., 1998). In some it is unclear whether they were included or not. In the studies that did include people with aphasia, aphasia often resulted in missed assessments (Ebrahim et al., 1986; Kwa et al., 1996; Wilkinson et al., 1997). Alternatively, proxy respondents were used (e.g., Astrom et al., 1992a; de Haan et al., 1995). Analysing proxy-reported HRQL findings alongside self-reported findings is questionable as quality of life is regarded as a highly subjective concept. The use of proxies is always less preferable than self-reports and the nature of HRQL may mean that the validity of proxy reports is further compromised. In some studies, no information is provided on how people with aphasia coped with the whole procedure (Bethoux, Calmels, & Gautheron, 1999; Foster & Young, 1996; King, 1996; Lofgren et al., 1999). This is problematic as it is anticipated that they would require at least some modification of the testing materials and special skills on behalf of the interviewer in order to give their experience of stroke. The validity of these assessments is therefore in doubt.

Another methodological challenge is that methods of assessing HRQL vary. Researchers have used a single Visual Analogue Scale (e.g., Kwa et al., 1996) to measure HRQL; an interview (e.g., Lawrence & Christie, 1979); generic scales like the Nottingham Health Profile (e.g., Wilkinson et al., 1997), the Sickness Impact Profile (de Haan et al., 1995; Hochstenbach, Donders, Mulder, vanLimbeek & Schoonderwaldt, 1996; Jonkman et al., 1998; Neau et al., 1998) and the Short Form-36 (Dorman, Dennis,

& Saundercock, 1999; Hackett, Duncan, Anderson, Broad, & Bonita, 2000; Wilkinson et al., 1997); or a battery of different tests (e.g., Angeleri et al., 1993). This methodological variation results in confusion as to what the concept of HRQL is supposed to reflect and what is the best way of measuring it.

A key conceptual challenge is that often the concept of quality of life is loosely defined or not defined at all (e.g., in Angeleri et al., 1993; Bethoux et al., 1999; Duncan et al., 1997; Kwa et al., 1996). In other studies HRQL/quality of life is not distinguished from related concepts, for example, it is expressed as life satisfaction (Ahlsio et al., 1984; Astrom et al., 1992a; Astrom et al., 1992b; Viitanen et al., 1988) or subjective well-being (Niemi et al., 1988). A few of the studies mentioned above did not set out to assess quality of life or HRQL *per se* but related concepts such as subjective well-being (Lofgren et al., 1999; Wyller et al., 1998), life satisfaction (Osberg et al., 1988), handicap (Clarke et al., 1999), and social and psychological effects of stroke (Ebrahim et al., 1986).

In the field of aphasiology, a number of studies have explored the *impact* of aphasia (e.g., more recently, Cruice, Worrall, & Hickson, 2000b; Hemsley & Code, 1996; Hoen, Thelander, & Worsley, 1997; LeDorze & Brassard, 1995; Lyon et al., 1997; Parr, Byng, & Gilpin, 1997; Sarno, 1997), rather than specifically the HRQL of people living with aphasia. Some of these studies have used measures such as the Ryff Psychological Well-being Scales (see Hoen et al., 1997) or the Psychological Well-being Index (see Lyon et al., 1997), which have not been tested extensively for their psychometric properties. Others have used semi-structured or in-depth interviewing techniques (LeDorze & Brassard, 1995; Parr et al., 1997). These studies give us useful information on issues related to the impact of aphasia. However, their methodology makes them hard to replicate in clinical practice and it is hard to draw comparisons between people with aphasia and other people living with stroke.

In summary, in recent years we have witnessed a proliferation of studies exploring the HRQL and related outcomes of people with stroke and aphasia. It remains a challenge to get a clear picture of the HRQL of people living with aphasia and the factors affecting it due to a number of conceptual and methodological issues (see also Cruice, Worrall, & Hickson, 2000a).

The current study's approach

The main aim of this study was to identify the main predictors of HRQL in people with chronic aphasia following stroke. Some of the challenges identified above were addressed in the current study in the following ways:

Conceptual clarity.   In this study HRQL is conceptualised as reflecting the impact of a health state on a person's ability to lead a fulfilling life (Bullinger et al., 1993). It incorporates the individual's subjective evaluation of his/her physical, mental/emotional, family, and social functioning (Berzon et al., 1993; de Haan et al., 1993; Hays et al., 1993).

Measurement approach: Potential for replication in clinical practice.   A viable way of investigating HRQL in people with aphasia in clinical practice is by use of a single HRQL measure. There is currently no single measure for the assessment of HRQL in people with aphasia. We have therefore modified the Stroke-specific Quality of Life Scale (SS-QOL, Williams, Weinberger, Harris, Clark & Biller, 1999), which is a patient-derived stroke-specific scale. The purpose of the modification was to make the measure communicatively accessible to people with aphasia and increase its content validity and acceptability with this population group (Hilari, 2000; Hilari & Byng, 2001). The resulting instrument is the Stroke and Aphasia Quality of Life Scale, 39-item version (SAQOL-39). SAQOL-39 has high acceptability, internal consistency, test–retest reliability and construct validity with people with chronic aphasia following stroke.[2]

Accessibility: Assessments used should be accessible to the population under study.   A speech and language therapist (SLT) experienced in working with people with aphasia carried out all the assessments in an interview format, in order to facilitate the understanding and communication of people with aphasia. All materials were shown to participants in an accessible format so that they could read the items while the interviewer said them. To facilitate participants' response, they had only to point to their responses. Materials used had been previously reviewed for their level of linguistic complexity. Although their content (in terms of meaning) remained unchanged to avoid invalidation, their presentation was modified to make them more communicatively accessible. In particular, few items were presented per page. Practice items were introduced at the beginning of each questionnaire to make sure the respondent understood the response format and what s/he had to do. Larger font was used (14–16pt) and key words were presented in bold (Hilari & Byng, 2001).

METHOD

Design

A cross-sectional design was adopted. A questionnaire-based interview was administered and data were collected on HRQL and potential predictors. The latter were demographic variables (age, sex, ethnic background, socioeconomic status, marital status, employment status); stroke and other health variables (type of stroke, time post-onset, and comorbidity); and other factors that have been associated with HRQL in people with stroke in other studies (emotional distress/depression, reduced activities, cognitive decline, aphasia, social support).

Participants

Participants were recruited as a clustered sample from two SLT service providers (NHS Trusts), one inner-city and one semi-rural, and a not-for-profit organisation for people with aphasia. All recruiting sites were in southeast England. The inclusion criteria were: aphasia due to a stroke, at least 1 year post-onset, no known pre-stroke history of severe cognitive decline or mental health problems, and living at home prior to the stroke.

Procedure

In the participating sites, review of SLT records was undertaken to identify eligible participants. Consent was obtained from eligible participants in writing at least 2 days after the main information on the project was given. All the participants were interviewed twice at home or in their SLT site by the main investigator, who administered all the questionnaires and assessments. Participants' aphasia was screened with the Frenchay

---

[2] The development and psychometric properties of the SAQOL-39 are fully described in Hilari (2002). Their publication in a peer-reviewed journal is planned for 2003. Further information and copies of the instrument can be requested of the first author.

Aphasia Screening Test (FAST) (Enderby, Wood, & Wade, 1987). If people scored less than 7/15 on the receptive domains of the FAST it was assumed, based on our previous research (Hilari & Byng, 2001), that they could not reliably understand the questionnaires that were used. On these occasions, with the participant's consent a proxy respondent was used (usually the spouse/partner or the main carer of the person with aphasia). These cases were excluded from the current analysis.

Measures

HRQL was assessed with the SAQOL-39, the aphasia adapted version of the SS-QOL. The SAQOL-39 asks questions about the effects of stroke and aphasia on people's lives that group into four domains: physical, psychosocial (including family and social issues), communication, and energy. Its response format is a 5-point scale ranging in the first part from "couldn't do it at all" to "no trouble at all" and in the second part from "definitely yes" to "definitely no".

Information on demographic, stroke-related, and comorbidity variables were collected from the participants' SLT notes. They were confirmed and supplemented through a short interview with the participants.

For emotional distress the General Health Questionnaire—12 item version (GHQ–12) (Goldberg, 1972) was used. The GHQ is a measure of distress that has been extensively used as a screening tool for psychiatric disorders. Its psychometric properties have been extensively tested (for reviews see Goldberg & Williams, 1988; Vieweg & Hedlund, 1983). It has also been used in stroke studies (e.g., Dennis, O' Rourke, Lewis, Sharpe, & Warlow, 2000; Dennis, O'Rourke, Slattery, Staniforth, & Warlow, 1997; Ebrahim et al., 1986).

To assess cognition, the Raven Coloured Progressive Matrices (RCPM) (Raven, 1962) was used. The RCPM uses non-verbal symbols to assess cognition, it does not require verbal responses from the respondents, and only minimal verbal instruction is necessary. As such it is, to the best of our knowledge, the most valid instrument for the assessment of cognition in people with language impairments. It has been used to explore cognitive decline in brain damage and aphasia (e.g., Villardita, 1985). The coloured rather than the standard matrices were preferred as they are considerably shorter, reducing respondent burden. Smits, Smit, van den Heuvel, and Jonker (1997) highlight two extra advantages of the RCPM. The matrices themselves are coloured large-print drawings, which are visible for older subjects with modestly impaired eyesight. Each part of the test starts with easy items, which is encouraging for the respondents as they can answer at least some of the items correctly.

Communication disability was assessed with the American Speech and Hearing Association Functional Assessment of Communication Skills for Adults (ASHA-FACS) (Frattali, Thompson, Holland, Wohl, & Ferketic, 1995). The ASHA-FACS asks about communicative activities that people with aphasia perform and whether they perform them independently or with assistance. Examples of items include requesting information of others, explaining how to do something, expressing feelings, and writing messages. It is rated by the SLT of the person with aphasia based on observations of this person or observations by others who are familiar with the person.

Participation in activities was explored with Frenchay Activities Index (FAI) (Wade, Legh-Smith, & Langton Hewer, 1985). The FAI is a measure of general (i.e., other than personal care) activities of stroke patients, which has been standardised on a sample of 976 stroke patients (seen just after the stroke, and at 3, 6, and 12 months post-onset). It includes in and outside the home activities, social and leisure activities, and an item on work.

Social support was assessed with the Social Support Survey (SSS) (Sherbourne & Stewart, 1991). The SSS assesses the perceived availability of four types of support (tangible, emotional/informational, social companionship, and affectionate support). It has a sound theoretical basis and good psychometric properties, which were tested on a group of chronically ill outpatients.

Data analysis

Multiple regression analysis (standard regression method, Tabachnik & Fidell, 2001) was used to assess the relative impact of a selected set of independent variables (IVs) on HRQL. We had a large number of potential predictors and a relatively modest sample size. This could challenge the viability of the regression analysis by reducing the cases to variables ratio. Tabachnick and Fidell (2001) suggest that for testing multiple correlation the simplest rule of thumb is $n \geqslant 50 + 8m$ (where m is the number of IVs). To reduce the number of variables that would enter the regression model, univariate analyses were initially undertaken between each IV and HRQL. One-way ANOVA, independent t-tests, and Pearson's product correlation coefficients were calculated depending on the nature of the IVs. The demographic, stroke, and health variables that were not significantly associated with HRQL in univariate analyses were not entered in the regression model. All other variables, i.e., emotional distress/depression, reduced activities, cognitive decline, aphasia, and social support, were included in the regression model. These variables are of theoretical interest as they have been implicated in previous research and their contribution to HRQL for people with aphasia needs to be assessed and better understood. They are also of greater interest to care providers as they may be addressed in rehabilitation and be subject to intervention. All analyses were performed with SPSS 10.0 for Windows (SPSS Inc., 1999).

RESULTS

Participants

A total of 116 eligible participants were identified and were asked to take part in the study. Of these, 95 people (82%) agreed to take part. No further information is available on the 21 people who did not take part as we did not have their consent for their records to be reviewed. Of the 95 people who took part in the study, 12 had such severe language problems (FAST receptive score < 7/15) that they were unable to self-report on the questionnaires that were used. For those participants proxy respondents were used and their results will be analysed separately in another study.

Table 1 details the characteristics of the remaining 83 participants. The majority were male (62.7%) and they ranged in age from 21 to 92 (mean 61.67 ± 15.47). About 43% were over 66 years old and 15.7% were between 21 and 45. The majority of the sample were white (78.3%) and married/had a partner (62.6%). Although almost 56% of the sample were of working age (≤ 65) only 6% were involved in some type of work (part-time or voluntary work and students). No participants were in full-time work. Participants' socioeconomic class was determined according to the new social classification system proposed by the Office of National Statistics (Rose & O' Reilly, 1997), which is based on occupation. Participants were classified according to their last occupation before the stroke, using the collapsed version of the socioeconomic classification (SEC).

TABLE 1
Characteristics of the participants

Characteristics	N = 83	Percent
Gender		
Female	31	37.3
Male	52	62.7
Age		
Mean (SD)	61.67 (15.47)	
Range	21–92	
21–45	13	15.7
46–65	34	41
66+	36	43.4
Stroke type		
Ischaemic	36	43.4
Haemorrhagic	16	19.3
Unknown	31	37.3
Time post-onset		
Mean in years (SD)	3.5 (3.09)	
Range	1y 1m–20y 10m	
1–2 years post-onset	26	31.3
2–4 years post-onset	31	37.3
4+ years post-onset	26	31.3
Comorbidity		
None or one comorbid condition	34	41
Two or more comorbid conditions	49	59
Ethnic group		
Asian	7	8.4
Black	11	13.3
White	65	78.3
Marital status		
Married	42	50.6
Has partner	10	12
Single	14	16.9
Divorced or spouse died	17	20.5
Socioeconomic status (revised collapsed SEC)		
Professionals/senior managers	23	27.7
Associate professional/junior managers	6	7.2
Other admin. and clerical workers	13	15.7
Own account non-professional	5	6
Supervisors, technicians and related workers	11	13.5
Intermediate workers	9	10.8
Other workers	12	14.5
Never worked/other inactive	4	4.8
Employment status		
Retired before the stroke	31	37.3
Inactive because of the stroke	47	56.6
Some p/t or voluntary work	3	3.6
Students	2	2.4

According to this criterion, approximately 35% were professionals and managers, 35% were other administrative and clerical workers, or own account non-professional and supervisors, or technicians and related workers, 25% were intermediate or other workers, and 5% had never worked.

Univariate analyses

HRQL as measured by the SAQOL-39 was normally distributed (Kolmogorov-Smirnov test ns at $p \leqslant .2$) with a mean(SD) of 3.27(.7) and a median of 3.26 and scores ranging from 1.72 to 4.46. Univariate analyses were used to assess the relations between HRQL and demographic, stroke-related, comorbidity, and other variables.

Demographic variables. The only demographic variable that was significantly correlated with HRQL was age ($r = -.27$, $p < .05$), with increased age associated with poorer HRQL. Gender, ethnic background, marital/relationship status, socioeconomic status, and employment status were not significantly associated with HRQL in this group of people with aphasia. These variables were not included in further analyses.

Stroke-related and other health variables. The stroke variables explored in this study (type of stroke and time post-onset) were not significantly associated with the participants' HRQL. Comorbidity was significantly and negatively correlated with HRQL ($r = -.25$, $p < .05$), with more comorbid conditions resulting in poorer HRQL. This variable was included in the subsequent multiple regression analysis.

Other variables. Descriptive statistics on the measures of depression/emotional distress (GHQ-12), level of activities (FAI), communication disability (ASHA-FACS), cognitive level (RCPM), and social support (SSS) are presented in Table 2.

Participants' scores on these measures were correlated with their HRQL (SAQOL-39) scores. All correlations were positive (wherever necessary scores were re-coded so that in all instruments high scores were indicative of good outcomes/function and low scores were indicative of poor outcome/function). The total scores were used for the FAI. There was one item in the FAI that asked about gardening and was not applicable to 30% of the respondents who did not have a garden. Missing data were imputed for each case, using the case's mean. The average of the ASHA-FACS and the SSS were used as recommended by the authors. The RCPM scores were converted to Standard Progressive Matrices (SPM) grades (Raven, Raven, & Court, 2000). The SPM grades range from 1–5 and they represent

TABLE 2
Descriptive statistics for ASHA-FACS, FAI, GHQ-12, SPM grade, and SSS

	ASHA-FACS	FAI	GHQ-12	SPM grade	SSS
N Valid	83	83	83	82	83
Missing	0	0	0	1	0
Mean	5.78	21.34	8.86	2.61	3.69
Median	5.95	22	10	2	3.89
Std. Deviation	.89	9.88	3.17	.91	.9547
Range	3.96	38	12	4	3.89
Minimum	2.99	3	0	1	1.11
Maximum	6.95	41	12	5	5.00

TABLE 3
Correlations of SAQOL-39 with GHQ-12, FAI, ASHA-FACS, SPM grade, and SSS

SAQOL-39	GHQ-12	FAI	ASHA-FACS	SPM grade	SSS
Pearson's correlation (r)	.53**	.58**	.46**	.27*	.19
Sig. (two-tailed)	.000	.000	.000	.014	.080
N	83	83	83	82	83

** Correlation significant at the .01 level (2-tailed).
* Correlation significant at the .05 level (2-tailed).

percentile ranks. SPM grades were also re-coded so that 5 was "intellectually superior", at or above the 95th percentile and 1 was "intellectually impaired", at or below the 5th percentile. Table 3 presents the results of these correlations.

The results suggest that HRQL was significantly poorer in people with high emotional distress ($p < .01$), high communication disability ($p < .01$), low activity level ($p < .01$), and low cognitive level ($p < .05$). High levels of social support were somewhat associated with better HRQL (the results approached significance with $p = .08$). All these variables were entered in the subsequent multiple regression analysis.

Multiple regression analysis

Multiple regression analysis was performed to assess the relationship between the dependent variable (DV) HRQL as expressed by the SAQOL-39 mean scores and correlated IVs. The standard method was used, where all IVs are entered in the regression equation at once. This way, each IV is evaluated in terms of what it adds to the prediction of the DV that is different from the predictability afforded by all other IVs. IVs were age, number of comorbid conditions, the GHQ-12, the FAI, the ASHA-FACS, the SPM grade, and the SSS.

Evaluation of the regression assumptions indicated that no transformation of variables was necessary. The residuals (differences between obtained and predicted DV scores) were normally distributed and the assumptions of homoscedasticity and linearity were met. The errors of prediction (residuals) were independent of one another (*Durbin-Watson* test of independence of errors = 2.09). Multicollinearity among IVs was not a problem: all tolerance values were > .2 (Menard, 1995). There were no outliers among IVs and on the DV: there were no particularly influential cases (maximum *Cook's distance* = .16, i.e., there were no values > 1); the average leverage $((m + 1)/n)$ (where m is the number of IVs) was 0.09 and the maximum *centered leverage* was .275 which is below $(3(m + 1)/n)$ as recommended by Stevens (1992); using a $p < .001$ criterion for *Mahalanobis distance*, there were no multivariate outliers among the cases (max = 22.304 < critical χ^2 for 7df at 24.322).

Table 4 displays a summary of the regression model. The overall model accounted for 51% of the variance (adjusted) in the SAQOL-39 scores. R for regression was significantly different from zero, with $F(7, 74) = 13.260$, $p < .001$.

Inspection of the B coefficients showed that emotional distress (GHQ-12) $t(74) = 3.81$, $p < .001$, activity level (FAI) $t(74) = 3.52$, $p \geqslant .001$, communication disability (ASHA-FACS) $t(74) = 2.15$, $p < .05$, and comorbidity $t(74) = -2.48$, $p < .05$, were significant predictors of HRQL (SAQOL-39). Three variables—cognition (SPM grade), social support (SSS), and age—were not significant predictors. Inspection of the 95% con-

TABLE 4
Summary of standard multiple regression analysis of the relation of HRQL with correlated predictors

Predictors	Adjusted R^2	R^2 Change	B	β	t
(Constant)			.63		1.09
ASHA			.18	.22	2.15*
FAI			2.531E-02	.36	3.52**
GHQ-12			7.823E-02	.35	3.81**
	.51***	.56***			
SPM grade			3.430E-02	.04	.51
SSS			4.563E-02	.06	.71
Cormobidity			−.30	−.21	−2.48*
Age			4.869E-03	.11	1.17

Dependent Variable: SAQOL-39 mean.
*** $p < .001$; ** $p < .01$; * $p < .05$.

fidence intervals for the IVs showed that for these three variables the confidence intervals included zero. This is further evidence that these three variables may weaken the overall model, as in some samples they have a negative relationship with HRQL and in others they have a positive relationship. For example, low cognitive level (as measured by the RCPM) was associated with good HRQL in some cases and poor HRQL in others.

A second regression analysis was run including only the significant predictors (i.e., emotional distress, activity level, communication disability, and comorbidity). In this model all the assumptions were met including the recommended cases-to-variables ratio where $n \geqslant 50 + 8m$, $n \geqslant 50 + (8.4)$, $n \geqslant 82$, and here $n \geqslant 83$. This model accounted for 52% of the variance (adjusted) in the SAQOL-39 scores. R for regression was significantly different from zero, with $F(4, 78) = 23.37$, $p < .001$. B coefficients showed that emotional distress (GHQ-12) $t(78) = 4.62$, $p < .001$, activity level (FAI) $t(78) = 3.40$, $p = .001$, communication disability (ASHA-FACS) $t(78) = 2.29$, $p < .05$, and comorbidity $t(78) = -2.18$, $p < .05$, were all significant predictors of HRQL (SAQOL-39).

In summary, high emotional distress, low activity level, high communication disability, and high comorbidity were significant predictors of poorer HRQL. These variables accounted for 52% of the variance of the SAQOL-39.

DISCUSSION

This study explored the main predictors of HRQL in people with chronic aphasia after stroke. One of the main strengths of this study lies in its design, which allowed 83 people with aphasia to self-report on the impact of stroke and aphasia on their lives. It highlights that careful selection of materials and mode of administration can ensure inclusion of people with communication disability in stroke studies. To the best of our knowledge this is the largest study of HRQL in people with aphasia in Britain.

Main findings

Of all eligible participants identified, 82% took part in the study. This high response rate indicates that our sample was representative of the population targeted. Physical disabilities and reduced level of activities have been repeatedly identified as among the main predictors of quality of life after stroke. High emotional distress and depression have also been repeatedly associated with reduced HRQL in people with stroke and aphasia. Our findings show a similar pattern with the subgroup of people living with aphasia after stroke and emphasise the potential importance of these aspects for effective service provision. In particular, our results highlight the importance of both identifying and then providing services to people experiencing emotional distress, as it continues to be a problem impacting on quality of life even in the long term after the stroke. However, a caveat here is that identifying that emotional distress is a significant predictor for quality of life does not necessarily mean that service providers should add assessing emotional distress to the battery of measures they implement. Asking people to reveal these kinds of problems is probably unethical unless something is going to be done with the information obtained, such as offering appropriate services or timely onward referral.

Services addressing the emotional distress that people with aphasia are dealing with are often not available routinely. The clear link with HRQL demonstrated here suggests that it should have a higher priority in service provision. Evidence suggests, however, that this need not necessarily be through implementing full-blown psychological therapies, for example, but could also be addressed through incorporation of work on self-esteem and confidence building alongside other therapies (e.g., Pound, Parr, Lindsay, & Woolf, 2000), or modification of attitude and behaviour by healthcare staff and carers, which can affect patients' motivation for and response to rehabilitation (Maclean, Pound, Wolfe, & Rudd, 2000; Parr et al., 1997).

The majority of stroke studies that included people with aphasia have concluded that the HRQL of people with aphasia was not significantly different from that of people living with the effects of stroke without aphasia. In the present study the impact of severity of communication disability on HRQL was assessed. We measured communication disability with the ASHA-FACS. The ASHA-FACS correlate highly with measures of aphasia language impairment, such as the Western Aphasia Battery (Kertesz, 1982) ($r = .76$, $p < .05$) (Frattali et al., 1995) and the FAST ($r = .79$, $p < .01$) (Hilari, 2002). Severity of communication disability (as measured by the ASHA-FACS) was a significant predictor of HRQL with higher communication disability resulting in poorer quality of life. This was despite the fact that the majority of our participants had high scores on the ASHA-FACS, i.e., indicative of mild communication disability (67.5% scored at or above 6, with scores ranging from 1 to 7). These findings are similar to the Kwa et al. (1996) study where 38% of the subjects had aphasia (measured with the Boston Diagnostic Aphasia Examination; Goodglass & Kaplan, 1983). Severity of aphasia was a significant predictor of quality of life despite the fact that data from the people with most severe aphasia were not included in the analysis (25% of their subjects could not complete the quality of life assessment due to communication problems).

A number of methodological issues may explain why aphasia was not a significant predictor of HRQL in other stroke studies. In some studies aphasia resulted in missed assessments (Angeleri et al., 1993; Ebrahim et al., 1986; Wilkinson et al., 1997). In other studies proxy respondents were used instead of the person with aphasia (Astrom et al., 1992a; Astrom et al., 1992b; de Haan et al., 1995; Neau et al., 1998; Tuomilehto et al., 1995). Studies on agreement between self-report and proxy respondents have found that there is considerable disagreement in rating functional abilities (Knapp & Hewison, 1999) and quality of life (Sneeuw, Aaronson, de Haan, & Limburg, 1997) after stroke. Hence, we believe it is advisable to analyse proxy data separately from self-report data. Lastly, in the remaining reviewed studies that included people with aphasia quite complex instruments were used to measure quality of life. These included the Ferrans and Powers quality of life index (Ferrans & Powers, 1985) in King (1996), the Philadelphia Geriatric Center Morale Scale (PGCMS, Lawton, 1975) in Lofgren et al. (1999), the Reintegration to Normal Living Index (RNLI, Wood-Dauphinee, Opzoomer, Williams, Marchant, & Spitzer, 1988) in Bethoux et al. (1999) and a 45-item questionnaire in Niemi et al. (1988). None of these studies gives any information on how people with aphasia managed these complex instruments. The validity of these assessments is questioned, as people with aphasia may have not understood at least some of the items or may have not been able to express their responses with precision.

Cognitive level was not a significant predictor of HRQL in our sample. Our findings agree with those of one study that specifically investigated the role of cognitive decline on quality of life after stroke (Kwa et al., 1996). These authors used the CAMCOG to measure cognition, which is part of the Cambridge Examination for Mental Disorders of the Elderly (CAMDEX; Roth et al., 1986). They indicated that people with aphasia were helped if needed with gestures and pointing. They concluded that cognitive decline was not a significant predictor of quality of life after stroke.

A few studies have associated cognitive decline with reduced quality of life after stroke (Clarke et al., 1999; Jonkman et al., 1998; Niemi et al., 1988). In the last two of these studies cognition was assessed with the Wechsler Adult Intelligence Scale (WAIS) and the Wechsler Memory Scale (WMS), which rely heavily on language. For people with aphasia, it is unclear whether such instruments measure language or cognitive skills. The third study (Clarke et al., 1999) did not attempt to differentiate between aphasia and cognitive decline. Rather the authors measured "cognitive disability" with the communication and cognition sub-scales of the Functional Independence Measure (FIM; Keith, Granger, Hamilton, & Sherwin, 1987). Such assessments will tend to identify people with aphasia as also having cognitive decline. The conclusion, therefore, that cognitive decline affects quality of life may well mask the effect of aphasia on quality of life. The results of the current study did not find a significant effect of cognitive decline on HRQL and may reflect the adaptation of measures to make them as accessible as possible to people with aphasia.

A number of studies have found that aspects of social support seem to affect quality of life after stroke (Astrom et al., 1992a; Astrom et al., 1992b; King, 1996; Osberg et al., 1988; Viitanen et al., 1988; Wyller et al., 1998). The absence of association between social support and HRQL in this sample of people with chronic aphasia may be related to the distribution of the social support scores. The SSS scores range from 1 to 5 with high scores indicating high social support, and in our sample the median was 3.9 and the mean 3.7. Only 12% of the participants scored 1 or 2 in this scale compared to 66.3% who scored 4 or 5. The fact that our sample had high levels of support may account, at least partly, for the lack of a significant association between social support and HRQL. Still, this lack of association may indeed be a true finding. In a related area, Robinson, Murata, and Shimoda (1999) found that during the first few weeks after stroke perceived social support was highly associated with depression whereas during the chronic period (12- or 24-month follow-up) this association was not significant, and other factors like financial security, living arrangements, and work experience were more pertinent.

The number of comorbid conditions was a significant predictor of HRQL in the regression analysis, whereas age was not. There was a tendency for older people to have more comorbid conditions ($r = .37$, $p < .001$), which seems to indicate that it is not age itself that leads to reduced quality of life but rather the increased health problems that it may bring with it.

Future research

Future studies could use the SAQOL-39 with stroke survivors with and without aphasia. This would allow for direct comparisons between different stroke groups. It would enable us to understand better the impact of aphasia as opposed to the impact of stroke and aphasia that was measured in this study.

More research is needed in the area of HRQL outcomes in severe aphasia using a range of methodologies. We will explore our findings on HRQL in people with severe aphasia using proxy respondents. Alternative methodologies may include qualitative techniques like participant and non-participant observation. However, all of these approaches are methodologically challenging. HRQL is generally defined as a subjective phenomenon. This makes it hard to observe without making value judgements that link the observed behaviour to the assumed subjective perception. This is problematic for measurement.

Further work is also needed to investigate the inter-relationship between communication disability, emotional distress, and activity level, and how they interact to affect HRQL. Longitudinal cohort studies could be used to unravel cause and effect relationships.

Future studies could also investigate the influence of social support on quality of life in aphasia. Using a combination of different support indicators such as social network (e.g., number of friends and relatives, contact with friends and relatives, group membership) and perceived support (e.g., the SSS) may help explore whether there are any effects that were not identified in the current investigation.

Summary and conclusion

The HRQL of people living with long-term aphasia after stroke is significantly affected by their emotional distress, their activity level, the severity of their communication disability, and their overall health. Service providers need to take these factors into account when planning and implementing interventions aimed at improving people's quality of life. Long-term services to people with aphasia can address emotional health, and enable participation in someone's immediate social context and in the community and society more generally (Byng, Pound, & Parr, 2000, Pound et al., 2000), and engage with the factors that contribute to communication disability.

REFERENCES

Ahlsio, B., Britton, M., & Murray, V. (1984). Disablement and quality of life after stroke. *Stroke, 15*, 886–890.

Angeleri, F., Angeleri, V. A., Foschi, N., Giaquinto, S., & Nolfe, G. (1993). The influence of depression, social activity, and family stress on functional outcome after stroke. *Stroke, 24*, 1478–1483.

Astrom, M., Adolfsson, R., Asplund, K., & Astrom, T. (1992a). Life before and after stroke. Living conditions and life satisfaction in relation to a general elderly population. *Cerebrovascular Disease, 2*, 28–34.

Astrom, M., Asplund, K., & Astrom, T. (1992b). Psychosocial function and life satisfaction after stroke. *Stroke, 23*, 527–531.

Berzon, R., Hays, R. D., & Shumaker, S. A. (1993). International use, application and performance of health-related quality of life instruments. *Quality of Life Research, 2*, 367–368.

Bethoux, F., Calmels, P., & Gautheron, V. (1999). Changes in the quality of life of hemiplegic stroke patients with time: A preliminary report. *American Journal of Physical Medicine and Rehabilitation, 78*, 19–23.

Bullinger, M., Anderson, R., Cella, D., & Aaronson, N. K. (1993). Developing and evaluating cross cultural instruments: From minimum requirements to optimal models. *Quality of Life Research, 2*, 451–459.

Byng, S., Pound, C., & Parr, S. (2000) Living with aphasia: Frameworks for therapy interventions. In I. Papathanasiou (Ed.), *Acquired neurological communication disorders: A clinical perspective.* London: Whurr Publishers.

Clarke, P. J., Black, S. E., Badley, E. M., Lawrence, J. M., & Williams, J. I. (1999). Handicap in stroke survivors. *Disability and Rehabilitation, 21,* 116–123.

Cruice, M., Worrall, L., & Hickson, L. (2000a). Quality of life measurement in speech pathology and audiology. *Asia Pacific Journal of Speech, Language and Hearing, 5,* 1–20.

Cruice, M., Worrall, L., & Hickson, L. (2000b). Quality of life for people with aphasia: Performance and usability of quality of life assessments. *Asia Pacific Journal of Speech, Language and Hearing, 5,* 85–91.

de Haan, R., Horn, J., Limburg, M., Van der Meulen, J., & Bossuyt, P. (1993). A comparison of five stroke scales with measures of disability, handicap, and quality of life. *Stroke, 24,* 1178–1181.

de Haan, R. J., Limburg, M., Van der Meulen, J. H. P., Jacobs, H. M., & Aaronson, N. K. (1995). Quality of life after stroke: Impact of stroke type and lesion location. *Stroke, 26,* 402–408.

Dennis, M., O'Rourke, S., Lewis, S., Sharpe, M., & Warlow, C. (2000). Emotional outcomes after stroke: Factors associated with poor outcome. *Journal of Neurology, Neurosurgery and Psychiatry, 68,* 47–52.

Dennis, M., O'Rourke, S., Slattery, J., Staniforth, T., & Warlow, C. (1997). Evaluation of a stroke family care worker: Results of a randomised controlled trial. *British Medical Journal, 314,* 1071.

Dorman, P., Dennis, M., & Sandercock, P. (1999). How do scores on the EuroQol relate to scores on the SF-36 after stroke. *Stroke, 30,* 2146–2151.

Duncan, P. W., Samsa, G. P., Weinberger, M., Goldstein, L. B., Bonito, A., Witter, D. M., Enarson, C., & Matchar, D. (1997). Health status of individuals with mild stroke. *Stroke, 28,* 740–745.

Ebrahim, S., Barer, D., & Nouri, F. (1986). Use of the Nottingham Health Profile with patients after a stroke. *Journal of Epidemiology and Community Health, 40,* 166–169.

Enderby, P., Wood, V., & Wade, D. (1987). *Frenchay Aphasia Screening Test.* Windsor, UK: NFER-Nelson.

Ferrans, C., & Powers, M. (1985). Quality of Life Index: Development and psychometric properties. *Advances in Nursing Science, 8,* 24.

Foster, A., & Young, J. (1996). Specialist nurse support for patients with stroke in the community: A randomised control trial. *British Medical Journal, 312,* 1642–1646.

Frattali, C. M., Thompson, C. K., Holland, A. L., Wohl, C. B., & Ferketic, M. M. (1995). *Functional assessment of communication skills for adults.* Rockville, MD: American Speech and Hearing Association.

Frey, W. D. (1984). Functional assessment in the 1980s: A conceptual enigma, a technical challenge. In A. S. Halpern & M. J. Furher (Eds.), *Functional assessment in rehabilitation.* Baltimore: Brookes.

Goldberg, D. P. (1972). *The detection of psychiatric illness by questionnaire.* London: Oxford University Press.

Goldberg, D. P., & Williams, P. (1988). *A user's guide to the General Health Questionnaire (GHQ).* Oxford: NFER-Nelson.

Goodglass, H., & Kaplan, E. (1983). *The assessment of aphasia and related disorders.* Philadelphia: Lea & Febiger.

Hackett, M. L., Duncan, J. R., Anderson, C. S., Broad, J. B., & Bonita, R. (2000). Health-related quality of life among long-term survivors of stroke. Results from the Auckland Stroke Study, 1991–1992. *Stroke, 31,* 440–447.

Hays, R. D., Anderson, R., & Revicki, D. (1993). Psychometric considerations in evaluating health-related quality of life measures. *Quality of Life Research, 2,* 441–449.

Hemsley, G., & Code, C. (1996). Interactions between recovery in aphasia, emotional and psychosocial factors in subjects with aphasia, their significant others and speech pathologists. *Disability and Rehabilitation, 18,* 567–584.

Hilari, K. (2000). Modification of the Stroke-Specific Quality of Life Scale for people with aphasia. *Quality of Life Research, 9,* 285(abstract).

Hilari, K. (2002). *Assessing health related quality of life in people with aphasia.* Unpublished doctoral dissertation, City University, London.

Hilari, K., & Byng, S. (2001). Measuring quality of life in aphasia: The Stroke-Specific Quality of Life Scale. *International Journal of Language and Communication Disorders, 36,* 86–91.

Hochstenbach, J. B., Donders, A. R., Mulder, T., van Limbeek, J., & Schoonderwaldt, H. (1996). Many chronic problems in CVA patients at home. *Ned Tijdschr Geneeskd, 140,* 1182–1186.

Hoen, B., Thelander, M., & Worsley, J. (1997). Improvement in psychological well-being of people with aphasia and their families: Evaluation of a community-based programme. *Aphasiology, 11,* 681–691.

Jonkman, E. J., de Weerd, A. W., & Vrijens, N. L. (1998). Quality of life after a first ischemic stroke. Long-term developments and correlations with changes in neurological deficit, mood and cognitive impairment. *Acta Neurologica Scandinavica, 98,* 169–175.

Keith, R. A., Granger, C. V., Hamilton, B. B., & Sherwin, F. S. (1987). The functional independence measure: A new tool for rehabilitation. In M. G. Eisenberg & R. C. Grzesiak (Eds.), *Advances in clinical rehabilitation* (pp. 6–18). New York: Springer.

Kertesz, A. (1982). *Western Aphasia Battery.* New York: Grune & Stratton.

King, R. B. (1996). Quality of life after stroke. *Stroke, 27,* 1467–1472.

Knapp, P., & Hewison, J. (1999). Disagreement in patient and carer assessment of functional abilities after stroke. *Stroke, 30,* 938

Kwa, V. I., Limburg, M., & de Haan, R. (1996). The role of cognitive impairment in the quality of life after ischaemic stroke. *Journal of Neurology, 243,* 599–604.

Lawrence, L., & Christie, D. (1979). Quality of life after stroke: A three-year follow-up. *Age and Ageing, 8,* 167–172.

Lawton, M. P. (1975). The Philadelphia Geriatric Centre Morale Scale: A revision. *Journal of Gerontology, 1,* 89.

Le Dorze, G., & Brassard, C. (1995). A description of the consequences of aphasia on aphasic persons and their relatives and friends, based on the WHO model of chronic diseases. *Aphasiology, 9,* 239–255.

Lofgren, B., Gustafson, Y., & Nyberg, L. (1999). Psychological well-being 3 years after stroke. *Stroke, 30,* 567–572.

Lyon, J. G., Cariski, D., Keisler, L., Rosenbek, J., Levine, R., Kumpula, J., Ryff, C., Coyne, S., & Blanc, M. (1997). Communication partners: Enhancing participation in life and communication for adults with aphasia in natural settings. *Aphasiology, 11,* 693–708.

Maclean, N., Pound, P., Wolfe, C., & Rudd, A. (2000) Qualitative analysis of stroke patients' motivation for rehabilitation. *British Medical Journal, 321,* 1051–1054.

Mayou, R., & Bryant, B. (1993). Quality of life in cardiovascular disease. *British Medical Journal, 69,* 460–466.

Menard, S. (1995). *Applied logistic regression analysis.* Thousand Oaks, CA: Sage.

Neau, J. P., Ingrand, P., Mouille-Brachet, C., Rosier, M. P., Couderq, C., Alvarez, A., & Gil, R. (1998). Functional recovery and social outcome after cerebral infarction in young adults. *Cerebrovascular Disease, 8,* 296–302.

NHS Executive (1996). *Promoting clinical effectiveness: A framework for action in and through the NHS.* Leeds, UK: Department of Health.

NHS Executive (1999). *Clinical governance in the new NHS.* London: NHS Executive Quality Management Branch.

Niemi, M. L., Laaksonen, R., Kotila, M., & Waltimo, O. (1988). Quality of life 4 years after stroke. *Stroke, 19,* 1101–1107.

Osberg, J. S., DeJong, G., Haley, S. M., Seward, M. L., McGinnis, G. E., & Germaine, J. (1988). Predicting long-term outcome among post-rehabilitation stroke patients. *American Journal of Physical Medicine and Rehabilitation, 67,* 94–103.

Parr, S., Byng, S., & Gilpin, S. (1997). *Talking about aphasia.* Buckingham, UK: Open University Press.

Patrick, D. L., & Erickson, P. (1993). Assessing health-related quality of life for clinical decision making. In S. R. Walker (Ed.), *Quality of life assessment: Key issues in the 1990s* (pp. 11–63). Dordrecht: Kluwer Academic Publishers.

Pound, C., Parr, S., Lindsay, J., & Woolf, C. (2000). *Beyond aphasia. Therapies for living with communication disability.* Bicester, UK: Speechmark Publishing Ltd.

Raven, J., Raven, J. C., & Court, J. H. (2000). *Standard Progressive Matrices.* Oxford: Oxford Psychologists Press.

Raven, J. C. (1962). *Coloured Progressive Matrices Sets A, Ab, B.* London: Lewis.

Robinson, R. G., Murata, Y., & Shimoda, K. (1999). Dimensions of social impairment and their effect on depression and recovery following stroke. *International Psychogeriatrics, 11,* 375–384.

Rose, D., & O'Reilly, K. (1997). *Constructing classes. Towards a new social classification for the UK.* Swindon, UK: ESRC/ONS.

Roth, M., Tyme, E., Mountjoy, C. Q., Hupert, F. A., Hendrie, A., Verma, S., & Goddard, R. (1986). CAMDEX: A standardised instrument for the diagnosis of mental disorders in the elderly with special reference to the early detection of dementia. *British Journal of Psychiatry, 149,* 698–709.

Royal College of Physicians (2000). *National clinical guidelines for stroke.* Prepared by The Intercollegiate Working Party for Stroke. London: RCP.

Sarno, M. T. (1997). Quality of life in aphasia in the first post-stroke year. *Aphasiology, 11,* 665–679.

Sherbourne, C. D., & Stewart, A. L. (1991). The MOS Social Support Survey. *Social Science and Medicine, 32,* 705–714.

Smits, C. H. M., Smit, J. H., van den Heuvel, N., & Jonker, C. (1997). Norms for an abbreviated Raven's Coloured Progressive Matrices in an older sample. *Journal of Clinical Psychology, 53,* 687–697.

Sneeuw, K. C. A., Aaronson, N. K., de Haan, R. J., & Limburg, M. (1997). Assessing quality of life after stroke. The value and limitations of proxy ratings. *Stroke, 28*, 1541–1249.

SPSS Inc. (1999). *SPSS Base 10.0 applications guide.* Chicago: SPSS Inc.

Stevens, J. P. (1992). *Applied multivariate statistics for the social sciences.* Hillsdale, NJ: Lawrence Erlbaum Associates, Inc.

Tabachnick, B. G., & Fidell, L. S. (2001). *Using multivariate statistics.* Boston, MA: Allyn & Bacon.

Tuomilehto, J., Nuottimaki, T., Salmi, K., Aho, K., Kotila, M., Sarti, C., & Rastenyte, D. (1995). Psychosocial and health status in stroke survivors after 14 years. *Stroke, 26*, 971–975.

Turner, R. R. (1990). Rehabilitation. In B. Spilker (Ed.), *Quality of life assessment in clinical trials* (pp. 247–267). New York: Raven.

Vieweg, B. W., & Hedlund, J. L. (1983). The General Health Questionnaire (GHQ): A comprehensive review. *Journal of Operational Psychiatry, 14*, 74–81.

Viitanen, M., Fugl-Meyer, K. S., Bernspaang, B., & Fugl-Meyer, A. R. (1988). Life satisfaction in long-term survivors after stroke. *Scandinavian Journal of Rehabilitation Medicine, 20*, 17–24.

Villardita, C. (1985). Raven's Colored Progressive Matrices and intellectual impairment in patients with focal brain damage. *Cortex, 21*, 627–634.

Wade, D. T., Legh-Smith, J., & Langton Hewer, R. (1985). Social activities after stroke: Measurement and natural history using the Frenchay Activities Index. *International Rehabilitation Medicine, 7*, 176–181.

Wenger, N. K., Mattson, M. E., Furberg, C. D., & Elison, J. (1984). Assessment of quality of life in clinical trials of cardiovascular therapies. *American Journal of Cardiology, 54*, 908–913.

Wilkinson, P. R., Wolfe, C. D. A., Warburton, F. G., Rudd. A. G., Howard, R. S., Ross Russell, R. W., & Beech, R. (1997). Longer term quality of life and outcome in stroke patients: Is the Barthel Index alone an adequate measure of outcome? *Quality in Health Care, 6*, 125–130.

Williams, L. S., Weinberger, M., Harris, L. E., Clark, D. O., & Biller, H. (1999). Development of a Stroke-Specific Quality of Life Scale. *Stroke, 30*, 1362–1369.

Wood-Dauphinee, S., & Williams, J. I. (1987). Reintegration to Normal Living as a proxy to quality of life. *Journal of Chronic Disease, 40*, 491–499.

Wood-Dauphinee, S. L., Opzoomer, M. A., Williams, J. I., Marchant, B., & Spitzer, W. O. (1988). Assessment of global function: The Reintegration to Normal Living Index. *Archives of Physical Medicine and Rehabilitation, 69*, 583–590.

World Health Organisation Quality of Life Assessment Group (1993). Study protocol for the World Health Organisation project to develop a quality of life assessment instrument, WHOQOL. *Quality of Life Research, 2*, 153–159.

Wyller, T. B., Holmen, J., Laake, P., & Laake, K. (1998). Correlates of subjective well-being in stroke patients. *Stroke, 29*, 363–367.

APHASIOLOGY, 2003, 17 (4), 383–396

Quality of life in aphasia:
Validation of a pictorial self-rating procedure

Barbara Engell, Bernd-Otto Hütter, Klaus Willmes, and Walter Huber

University of Technology (RWTH), Aachen, Germany

Methods & Procedures: Quality of life was assessed for stroke patients with aphasia in postacute and chronic stages by means of the Aachen Life Quality Inventory (ALQI), a German adaptation of the Sickness Impact Profile (SIP). A modified written version of the ALQI was given to relatives, and a newly developed pictorial version designed to minimise language demands was given to aphasic patients. Ratings of 24 patient–relative pairs were assessed.

Outcomes & Results: Overall the two versions were found to be highly parallel and internally consistent, and they could be separated equally well along physical and psychosocial dimensions. In addition to rating complaints, patients were asked to score the burden caused by them; high intercorrelations between complaints and burden were found. The physical subscore was influenced by presence and degree of hemiparesis, and the psychosocial subscore by patients' mood state as rated by the relatives. Age had an impact on relatives' ratings of language and cognition as well as on physical functions. Patients and relatives differed in rating of psychosocial and cognitive complaints. Relatives took a more functional perspective; patient ratings were more dependent upon degree and quality of the aphasic impairment.

Quality of life is a concept that is increasingly considered to be important for the assessment of rehabilitation (Flanagan, 1982; Orley & Kuyken, 1994; Spitzer, 1987). The notion of "quality of life" is used both in the sense of subjective feelings and attitudes, and in the sense of absence or presence of complaints resulting from disability or handicap (Aaronson, 1988; Allison, Locker, & Feine, 1997; Katz, 1987). Thus, when subjects are asked to rate their quality of life, it may be related to emotional states, to physical and psychosocial abilities, or to all of them.

In the context of neurological rehabilitation, physical and psychosocial abilities are often considered to be more specific and therefore more important than emotions in determining quality of life (de Haan, Aaronson, Limburg, Langton Hewer, & van Crevel, 1993). Quality of life ratings are used to complement the assessment of motor or cognitive performance as measures of rehabilitation outcome (de Haan, Limburg, van der Meulen, Jacobs, & Aaronson, 1995; Kim, Warren, Madill, & Hadley, 1999; King, 1996;

Address correspondence to: Walter Huber, PhD, Section of Neurolinguistics, Department of Neurology, University of Technology (RWTH), Pauwelsstrasse 30, D-52074 Aachen, Germany.
Email: huber@neuroling.rwth-aachen.de

This study was supported by a grant from the "Interdisciplinary Centre for Clinical Research – CNS" of the Medical Faculty of the Technical University (RWTH) Aachen. We would like to thank Irene Blume for her work in designing and drawing the pictures. Marc Brügmann guided parts of the statistical evaluation. Special thanks to Linda Worrall and Audrey Holland who helped us to improve the manuscript.

http://www.tandf.co.uk/journals/pp/02687038.html   DOI:10.1080/02687030244000734

Visser, 1996). There is an obvious need for rating of quality of life, given the fact that traditional neuropsychological test batteries do not directly measure the functional outcome of improved skills and capacities. In many patients, there is a gap between improved performance in the laboratory and persistence of problems in daily life.

Language impairment has long-lasting consequences for everyday communication and activity, and also hinders patients' abilities to evaluate and report on their situation. Concerns about reading and auditory comprehension have not explicitly been dealt with in quality of life studies on aphasia (Hoen, Thelander, & Worsley, 1997; Taylor Sarno, 1997). We therefore chose to develop a pictorial procedure for rating quality of life to minimise the influence of aphasia. We transformed an existing quality of life inventory—the modified German version of the Sickness Impact Profile (Bergner, Bobitt, Carter & Gilson, 1981; Hütter, 2001)—into a picture-based presentation.

In recent years, several analyses of both group and single case studies have emphasised the importance of evidence for the effectiveness of aphasia therapy (Enderby & Emerson, 1995; Pearson, 1995; Robey, 1994, 1998). There is ongoing debate about which kind of outcome measures are most appropriate. The choice ranges from fully standardised reliable aphasia batteries to experimentally developed tests that are tailored to the individual symptom complex. Many authors suggest that deficit-oriented measures should be complemented or even substituted for by measures of communicative functioning in real-life situations (e.g., Greener, Enderby, & Whurr, 2002). Another option is to ask caregivers and/or patients directly to estimate the type and amount of complaints or the degree of adaptation to the handicap. The validity of such ratings should be increased if parallel questionnaires are available.

In this study, we report on the development and validation of a new quality of life questionnaire for aphasia patients. Our main objective was to construct and validate a procedure that would allow for self-rating of aphasic patients in parallel to a proxy rating by caregivers. To keep the language demands low, a pictorial version for patients was developed that corresponded item by item to the caregivers' written version.

METHOD

Materials

We selected the Aachen Quality of Life Inventory (ALQI; Hütter, 2001; Hütter & Gilsbach, 1996; Hütter & Würtemberger, 1997), a German language adaptation of the Sickness Impact Profile (SIP; Bergner et al., 1981). The original SIP categories were reduced but the total score and two subscores were preserved.

Each item of the ALQI presents a statement of a physical or psychosocial complaint that is judged to be true or false by patients and by caregiving persons. The patient's self-rating version of the ALQI includes an additional three-step scale per item for weighting the burden of a complaint.

While the SIP was developed as a self-rating instrument for subjects with general physical health problems, the ALQI was specifically validated for brain-damaged patients after neurosurgical treatment ($n = 281$) as well as for their relatives ($n = 163$) (Hütter & Gilsbach, 1996). For both samples, the ALQI was demonstrated to have high internal consistency and high split-half reliability. The coefficients were above .90 for the total scale and above .80 for the two dimensions of the inventory, which grouped four physical and five psychosocial categories of 10 items each. The nine subscales attained high consistency and reliability with coefficients above .70. Furthermore, patients and relatives were highly correlated.

For the adaptation, the ALQI items were transformed into a pictorial version, to maximise aphasic patients' understanding of the verbal statements as well as to permit them to give nonverbal responses. Our aim was to develop an inventory that could be handled even by patients with severe language comprehension deficits. Figure 1 shows an example taken from the category "social interaction". All pictures are professionally rendered simple line-drawings. Statements represent an everyday-life situation exemplifying a typical psychosocial or physical problem of adults. Half of the depicted characters are female, half are male. As illustrated in Figure 1, a written phrase was added to each depicted situation expressing the core proposition in telegraphic style. When a new picture is shown, these headings are read aloud to the patient. Such multimodal input was intended to maximise patients' abilities to understand each item.

Additional simple pictograms permitted the patients to indicate their ratings. A forced choice format ("thumb up/down") combined with the written phrases "yes, that's true/ no, that's not true" (see Figure 1) was used. When a patient indicated yes, he or she was next asked to judge the degree of burden by making a choice between a neutral, a frowning, and a weeping face combined with the written emotional expressions "doesn't matter" ("*egal*"), "bad" ("*schlimm*"), "very bad" ("*sehr schlimm*").

Like the SIP, the ALQI in its original and in our new pictorial version allows for the calculation of physical and psychosocial subscores in addition to the total score. The subscores are derived from several sub-domains representing different categories of quality of life. To meet the special circumstances of patients with language disorders and possible associated cognitive dysfunctions, two more categories were added that contain specific aphasic and neuropsychological complaints. They are not included in the total

often alone

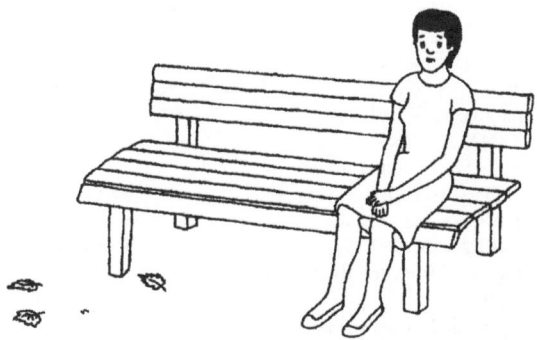

Figure 1. Item example from the category Social Interaction of the pictorial version of the Aachen Life Quality Inventory (ALQI).

score to allow comparison with ALQI and SIP ratings of nonaphasic patient groups. Table 1 lists all categories in the order in which they are presented. The total number of items is 117.

In a pilot study we asked 21 students of speech and language pathology to rate the degree of correspondence between the written and the pictorial version of the ALQI. Subjects indicated their ratings using a 5-point scale (5 indicating perfect and 1 indicating no correspondence). We obtained an overall mean of 3.7 (range 3.3–4.3) for the 11 categories. Thus, the two versions appeared to be sufficiently congruent to merit further study. Patients were given the pictorial version; relatives were assessed using the written version of the inventory. Scales for rating the burden of complaints were included only in the patients' version. Relatives were instructed to estimate the complaints of their aphasic partners (proxy rating). That is, they were asked to put themselves into the aphasic partner's shoes.

To control for patients' mood states, the depression subscale of the Profile of Mood State (POMS; McNair, Lorr, & Dropelman, 1971) was also given to the relatives. To assess the type and severity of aphasia, the Aachen Aphasia Test was used (AAT; Huber, Poeck, Weniger, & Willmes, 1983; Huber, Poeck, & Willmes, 1985).

Procedure

The study was conducted on the aphasia ward of the University Hospital in Aachen. On this 12-bed ward, patients are treated for 7 weeks. Besides an intensive programme of

TABLE 1
Design of the Aachen Quality of Life Inventory (ALQI)

Category/Example	Dimension	Number of items
• ACTIVITY	PSYCHOSOCIAL	10
e.g., sitting around half-asleep		
• MOVEMENT	PHYSICAL	10
e.g., standing up only with help		
• HOME MANAGEMENT	PHYSICAL	10
e.g., no heavy work around the house		
• SOCIAL INTERACTION	PSYCHOSOCIAL	10
e.g., being often alone		
• FAMILY RELATIONSHIP	PSYCHOSOCIAL	10
e.g., turning away from family members		
• AMBULATION	PHYSICAL	10
e.g., getting around in wheelchair		
• COMMUNICATION	PSYCHOSOCIAL	10
e.g., have difficulty speaking		
• LEISURE	PSYCHOSOCIAL	10
e.g., going out for entertainment less often		
• SELF-SUPPORT	PHYSICAL	10
e.g., need help with bathing		
• COGNITION		14
e.g., forgetting a lot		
• LANGUAGE		13
e.g., have difficulty finding words		

Categories are given in the order of examination; examples are taken from the pictorial version (translations from German).

speech and language therapy (9 full hours per week) (Huber, Springer, & Willmes, 1993; Poeck, Huber, & Willmes, 1989), patients are provided with physical therapy, neuropsychological training, psychosocial counselling, and medical check-ups. To be admitted, patients must be beyond the acute phase of illness and largely able to function independently.

Only patients who had been discharged from acute care at least 3 weeks before admission to the ward were assessed. During the first day on the ward, they were given the pictorial version of the ALQI with the instruction to judge their everyday life during the previous week at home. Assessment took place in a quiet room. The examiner sat on the opposite side of the table, read the headings aloud, and made sure that the patients answered each item. There was no time limit.

The written version of the ALQI was also given on the first day to the family member who accompanied the patient and who was familiar with his or her living conditions at home. Partners were asked to fill out both the written version of the ALQI and the POMS before they left the hospital.

Participants

The study included 26 patients and 24 partners. One relative chose not to participate and one patient lived alone. In 21 instances the written ALQI was filled out by the spouse, in 3 instances by other family members. The median age of the patients was 54 years (range 26–69), 9 patients were female and 17 male. Of these patients, 13 had less than 10 years formal education; formal education for the other 13 resulted in pre-university degrees ("*Abitur*"). Strokes were the cause of aphasia in all cases. The median duration of aphasia was 12 months (range 1–63). A total of 18 patients had right hemiparesis/hemiplegia, judged as severe in 8 cases and moderate to mild in 10 cases; 17 patients had non-fluent aphasia (8 global, 6 Broca's, and 3 non-classifiable aphasia), and 9 were fluent (1 Wernicke's, 1 amnesic, 1 transcortical-sensory, 4 non-classifiable, and 2 residual aphasia).

RESULTS

Comparison between patients' and relatives' ratings

The mean values for the 24 patient–relative pairs of ratings are shown in Figure 2. Similar mean numbers of complaints were found for patients and relatives on each scale. Means for the psychosocial and physical subscores as well as for the total score are almost identical. None of the differences was significant when multiple t-tests for dependent samples as well as Wilcoxon signed ranks tests were applied. Likewise, no significant differences were found for any of the individual categories (all p-values greater than .10) with the exception of activity and language. Relatives reported markedly more complaints than patients for language ($p = .04/.06$, t-test/Wilcoxon signed ranks test, two-tailed), but fewer for activity ($p = .08/.08$).

Among the physical categories, few complaints were found for self-support and movement, significantly more for ambulation and home management. Most likely this was because patients being admitted to the aphasia ward had to be able to function largely independently.

Among the psychosocial categories, few complaints were reported for activity, family relationships, and social interaction, significantly more for communication and leisure. Overall, the proportions of complaints were rather moderate with peaks around 50%. This

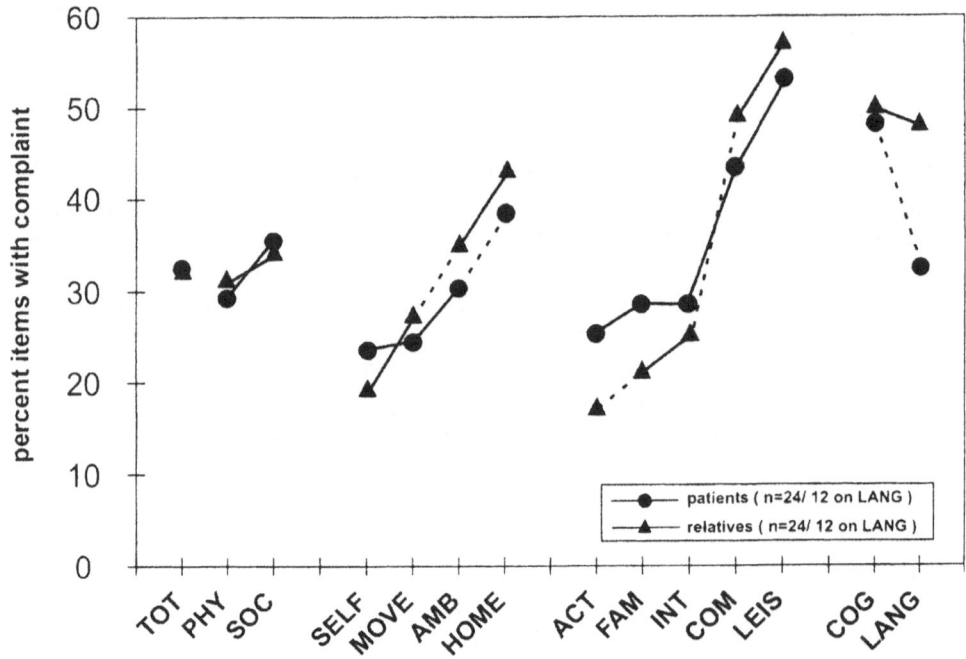

Figure 2. Mean percentages of complaints (*n* = 24 patient–relative pairs; due to a technical failure the ratings on Language were only registered from 12 relatives): dotted lines indicate significant differences between categories (*p* < .05, Wilcoxon signed ranks test, two-tailed).

was also true for the newly developed categories of cognition and language. Surprisingly, patients reported significantly fewer complaints on language than on cognition.

Next we computed correlation coefficients (see Table 2). The patient's and relative's ratings were significantly correlated for the total score and physical subscale, but not for the psychosocial subscale. High correlations were found for ambulation, self-support, moderate ones for leisure and activity.

Reliability and construct validity

We assessed the internal consistency of judgements on each category separately for patients and relatives (see Table 2). Given the small sample size, coefficients of .70 and higher were used to indicate sufficient consistency. As can be seen in Table 2, this level was reached for the total score and the two subscores as well as for most of the individual categories.

By means of nonmetric multidimensional scaling using the Smallest Space Analysis program (SSA; Borg, 1992; Lingoes, 1979), we assessed how well the categories could be grouped according to dimensions (physical versus psychosocial) and subjects (patients versus relatives). Based on intercorrelations, we obtained a two-dimensional spatial representation of all quality of life categories as judged by either patients or relatives. Categories being similar in rating are spatially close together. The result of the SSA is shown in Figure 3.

Overall, the categories are well separated according to whether they were rated by patients or relatives and whether they belonged to the psychosocial or the physical subscore. Roughly, the two-dimensional space can be divided into quadrants (Figure 3).

TABLE 2
Correlations and consistence

	No items	Correlations		Cronbach's alpha		Split-half reliability	
		r	r_s	patients	relatives	patients	relatives
Total score	90	.39*	.42*	.90	.94	.88	.93
Physical score	40	.64**	.66**	.90	.93	.69	.75
self-support	10	.52**	.65**	.89	.89	.82	.91
movement	10	.28	.21	.44	.79	.52	.75
ambulation	10	.75**	.73**	.76	.89	.83	.87
home management	10	.25	.29	.76	.87	.82	.86
Psychosocial score	50	.27	.26	.79	.91	.68	.77
activity	10	.31	.49*	.73	.82	.72	.81
family relationship	10	−.01	−.02	.51	.82	.65	.68
social interaction	10	.00	.05	.12	.68	.08	.84
communication	10	.13	.13	.69	.63	.74	.65
leisure	10	.43*	.47*	.63	.75	.62	.64
Cognition	14	−.09	−.10	.70	.73	.74	.80
Language[†]	13	.00	.06	.59	.70°	.34	.75°

Correlations between patients' and relatives' ratings ($n = 24$) and internal consistency of ratings ($n = 26$ patients, $n = 24/$[†]$n = 12$ relatives).
[†] Due to a technical failure only 12 relatives' ratings were registered for Language.
** $p < .01$, * $p < .05$ significantly different from zero, Pearson (r) and Spearman (r_s) correlation coefficients.

Relatives' ratings are clustered in the upper quadrants, patients' ratings in the lower; physical categories are on the right, psychosocial ones on the left.

Among the physical categories, relatives' and patients' ratings on ambulation (AMB in Figure 3), movement (MOVE), and self-support (SELF), are spatially adjacent, i.e., they are highly correlated. An exception is home management (HOME), which is judged differently by aphasic patients and their relatives.

Among the psychosocial categories, high agreement between patient's and relative's ratings was found only for leisure (LEIS), which appears to be more appropriately grouped with the physical than the psychosocial categories. On all other psychosocial categories, patients' and relatives' ratings are further apart than on the physical ones, i.e., they showed lower correlations. The newly developed categories of language (LANG) and cognition (COG) are spatially closer to the psychosocial than to the physical categories. As can be expected, patients' ratings on language (LANG) and on communication (COM) are closely related. (The relatives' ratings on language were not considered as we obtained only 12 reports due to a technical failure.)

Influence of control variables

Quality of life ratings can be influenced by several demographic and clinical factors. We considered the following:

- Gender: female vs male ($n = 9$ vs 17).
- Age: below vs equal/above median age of 54 years ($n = 11$ vs 15).
- Education: lower vs higher level ($n = 13$ vs 13).
- Duration of aphasia: less vs more than 12 months ($n = 12$ vs 14).

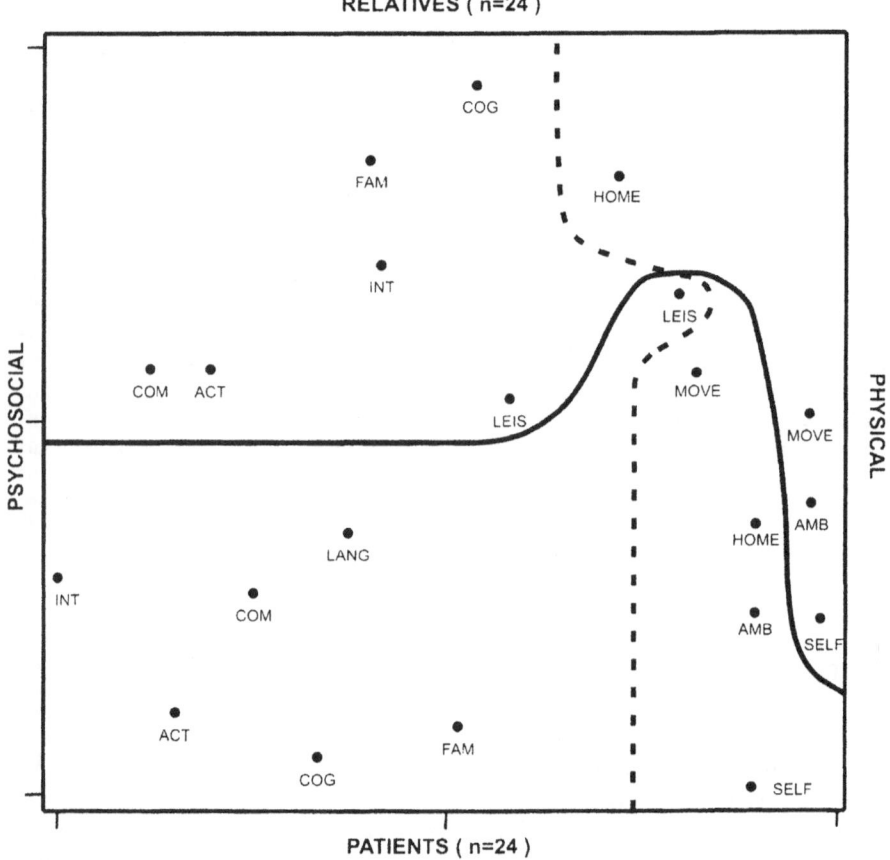

Figure 3. Smallest space analysis (SSA) for similarity in ratings (monotonicity coefficient μ_2, two dimensional solution, coefficient of alienation = 0.181).

- Speech output: fluent vs nonfluent (n = 9 vs 17) derived from AAT-ratings of syntax in spontaneous language (scores 0–2 were classified as nonfluent, scores 3–5 as fluent).
- Overall degree of language impairment: severe vs moderate to mild (n = 9 vs 17) derived from AAT norms on Token Test performance (smaller vs equal/greater percentile 38).
- Hemiparesis/hemiplegia: present vs absent (n = 18 vs 8).
- State of mood: depressive vs non-depressive (n = 14 vs 7) derived from relatives' ratings (3 out of 24 missing).

T-tests were used to assess the impact of these factors. For both patients and relatives, neither the total ALQI score nor the two subscores were significantly influenced by gender, educational level, or duration of aphasia. Age, however, had an impact, with significantly more physical complaints reported by and for older patients (p = .043 and .036). Partly this was due to the fact that 12 out of 15 older patients were hemiparetic, while only 6 out of 11 were younger ones. In addition, the older patients were judged by their partners as having significantly more complaints about limited cognitive capacities than younger patients (p = .031).

A significant impact was found for fluency of speech output, with nonfluent aphasics reporting significantly more complaints than fluent aphasics on the total score ($p = .006$) and the physical subscore ($p = .005$), and close to significantly more complaints on the psychosocial subscore ($p = .095$) and on the language category ($p = .069$), but not on the cognition category ($p = .118$). This was in part also related to the presence of severe and moderate paresis in all but two of the non-fluent aphasics ($n = 17$) as opposed to only three cases of mild to moderate paresis in the fluent aphasics ($n = 9$). In contrast to fluency, overall degree of language impairment as measured by the Token Test had no significant impact on quality of life ratings.

Not surprisingly, both the hemiparetic patients and their partners reported significantly more physical complaints than patients with no or with recovered movement disorders ($p = .001$).

On the other hand, patients who were judged by their realtives as being depressive indicated more complaints than non-depressive patients on the cognition category ($p = .023$). The relatives reported more psychosocial complaints for these depressive patients ($p = .025$).

Correlations between quality of life ratings and language performance

To assess further the impact of severity of aphasia, the ALQI ratings were correlated with performance scores of the AAT. We expected high negative correlations, i.e., poor performance should be correlated with high number of complaints (and vice versa). There was a striking difference between the ratings of the patients themselves and the ratings of their partners. Only the patients' ratings were as anticipated, whereas no significant correlations were found for the judgements of partners, except for written language, which was significantly correlated with physical complaints ($r_S = -.40$, $p < .05$ for difference from zero).

Regarding the judgements of the patients, their ALQI total score as well as their two subscores were significantly correlated with communicative and systematic failures in spontaneous language—occurrence of automatised elements, semantic, phonemic, and syntactic errors (r_S range $-.40$ to $-.63$, $p < .05/.01$ for difference from zero)—but not with articulation disorders (r_S range $-.10$ to $-.32$).

Among the AAT subtests, significant correlations of total and subscore were obtained for the expressive subtests—repetition, naming, written language (r_S range $-.39$ to $-.52$). For the receptive subtests (Token Test, comprehension), there was only one strong correlation; this was between the psychosocial subscore and performance on the Token Test ($r_S = -.50$).

Patients' burden score

The self-rating version of the ALQI also contained 3-point scales for weighting the burden of each complaint (2 = "very bad"; 0 = "doesn't matter"). For each ALQI variable a relative burden score was calculated, i.e., the average burden per complaint. Patients felt only moderately affected by their complaints; the average burden was 0.8 on the total core, 0.7 on the physical, and 0.8 on the psychosocial subscore.

As can be expected, number of complaints and burden scores were very highly correlated. All coefficients were close to .90 or above. Consequently, highest relative burden scores were found for those categories with the most complaints, i.e., leisure, communication, cognition, and language. On these categories about half of the items were judged to represent true complaints and they were given on the average moderate relative burden scores (between 0.8 and 1.1 per complaint on the 2-point scale). In contrast, fewer complaints were registered on all other dimensions and their burden scores varied in a lower range between 0.4 and 0.7. The categories with the fewest complaints—self-support and activity—also obtained the lowest ratios for burden per complaint.

The degree of depression as judged by relatives was not significantly correlated with the burden scores for any of the ALQI variables.

DISCUSSION

Psychometric properties

Overall we can conclude that the new versions of the ALQI appear to have sufficiently good psychometric properties for the study of quality of life in aphasia. As the sample size of 24 patient–relative pairs was small, the results of this study must be taken as preliminary. The items of the written and pictorial version were found to be parallel and internally consistent. Distinguishing a physical from a psychosocial dimension is empirically justified. The two new categories concerning language and cognition cluster together with the other psychosocial categories.

The original ALQI, which is an adaptation and modification of the SIP, was developed for the assessment of patients undergoing neurosurgery. All patients of the present study suffered from stroke and subsequent aphasia, being either in the postacute (> 1 month) or in the chronic (> 12 months) stage. The preliminary psychometric properties found in this study are quite comparable to those reported for the original ALQI (Hütter & Gilsbach, 1996) and the SIP (Bergner et al., 1981). Our new pictorial patients' version showed internal consistencies and intercorrelations that are very similar to those found for the written relatives' version. The pictorial version was specifically developed for aphasic patients to enable them to understand and respond to quality of life questions relatively free of language. Using pictorial information is indeed a valid and reliable technique for the assessment of quality of life in aphasia. Even scoring of a burden caused by the complaints could be easily undertaken by means of pictograms. The results show, however, that the ratings of complaint and burden were highly interrelated in the aphasic patients as a group.

Quantity and quality of the complaints

In previous studies using the SIP in stroke patients, *total complaint scores* ranged from 11% (Visser, 1996) to 23% (de Haan et al., 1995) and 25% (Granger, Cotter, Hamilton, & Fiedler, 1993), which is high compared to groups with other chronic disease (Damiano, 1996). In this study the average number of complaints was even higher, with approximately one in three of the items indicating complaints for both aphasic patients and their relatives. This relatively high proportion appears to be determined by the presence of aphasia. Life quality seems to be specifically affected by aphasia, even though with respect to the average complaint, the patients thought they were only moderately affected.

Considering the individual categories of each *subscore*, the profiles of patients and relatives ratings were almost identical. There was no general tendency for relatives to overrate the complaints of the patients as was suggested in previous studies (Taylor Sarno, 1997). When not only number of complaints but also correlations between ratings of patients and relatives were considered, individualised patterns were obtained.

Among the *physical categories*, there was an increase in number of complaints from self-support to home management, with movement and ambulation coming in between. In previous applications of the SIP, home management was also judged to be most deteriorated in post-stroke patients (Carod-Artal, Egido, González, & de Seijas, 2000; de Haan et al., 1995; Visser, 1996).

We found no significant differences in number of complaints between patients and relatives for any categories. Ratings were significantly correlated for self-support and ambulation, but not for movement and home management. Apparently, aphasic patients experienced difficulties in movement and managing their household that went unnoticed by relatives.

There were also differences between *psychosocial categories*. Low mean numbers of complaints were found for activity, family relationship, and social interaction (2–3 complaints per 10 items each) as opposed to almost twice as many complaints for communication and leisure. Similar degradations in such categories, except for communication, were reported for stroke survivors by Niemi, Laaksonen, Kotila, and Waltimo (1988) and Visser (1996). Leisure was closely associated with life satisfaction of stroke patients in a study by Parker, Gladman, and Drummond (1997). With respect to communication, Visser (1996) found surprisingly few complaints—however her sample included only a small number of aphasic patients.

In our study relatives reported more complaints than patients in the more affected psychosocial categories. The opposite was found for the less affected ones. Only for activity was the difference statistically significant. In contrast to the physical categories, correlations between the ratings of patients and relatives on other psychosocial categories were low. Being aphasic seems to be viewed differently by patients and relatives in relation to psychosocial aspects of everyday behaviour. For example, patients complained frequently about needing a rest, whereas withdrawing from family life was most likely to be a complaint reported by relatives.

For *language* and *cognition*, the judgements of patients and relatives were also different. Relatives reported significantly more complaints on language than did patients. They appeared to make more realistic judgements on kind and extent of language disorders. However, this interpretation is contradicted when ratings on language are compared to performance on the Aachen Aphasia Test (AAT). For patients, high correlations were found between language complaints and nearly every AAT measure. Most likely, they considered their language difficulties to be the primary source for their problems in memory, execution, and attention. Relatives viewed linguistic and cognitive difficulties as independent. They seem to take a more functional perspective, i.e., they perceive the aphasic difficulties in the context of possible achievements in everyday life, and less as a handicap in conveying ideas and emotions, the primary focus of the patients. As a consequence, the relatives attributed significantly more linguistic complaints to their aphasic partners than were reported by the patients themselves.

External factors

How good is the external validation of the two ALQI versions? To what extent was it possible to assess quality of life in conditions of aphasia independent of intervening demographic and clinical factors? Regarding gender, age, and education of the patients, only *age* had an impact. With increasing age of the patients, relatives reported more complaints about language and cognition. Apparently ageing enhances aphasia-related deficits as seen by caregivers. Interestingly, this was more pronounced for complaints about cognition than on language *per se*.

In addition, we found significantly more physical complaints reported for and by patients above 54 years, the median age of the sample. This was only in part determined by unequal distribution of motor disorders in the two subgroups. Distinguishing between severe, moderate to mild, and no hemiparesis, proportions of 5, 7, and 3 cases were obtained for the older subgroup ($n = 15$) and similar proportions of 3, 3, and 5 cases for the younger subgroup ($n = 11$). One possible explanation is that younger stroke patients and their relatives adapt to their physical handicap more efficiently and therefore have fewer complaints. Alternatively, with increasing age, physical handicaps are harder to bear.

Regardless of age, there was a strong and significant overall impact of *paretic disorders* on the number of physical complaints being reported by both patients and relatives. On average, about three times more complaints were obtained for hemiparetic than for non-hemiparetic patients. The total ALQI score was also affected, even though no significant difference was found for the psychosocial subscore.

The patient's *mood state* as rated by the relatives had a clear impact on the psychosocial score. Relatives showed high positive correlations between their psychosocial and depression ratings, and they reported almost twice as many psychosocial complaints for patients judged to be depressed than for those judged as non-depressed. Furthermore, the depressed patients themselves reported more cognitive complaints. In further studies momentary state of mood should be assessed when patients are asked to consider their quality of life. This can be investigated directly by using a pictorial mood scale such as that recently developed by Stern, Arruda, Hooper, Wolfner, and Morley (1997).

In contrast to Visser (1996), we did not find a significant impact of time post-onset. Finally, *type of aphasia* had an impact. Nonfluent patients reported more psychosocial and linguistic complaints than did patients who had fluent speech output. In contrast, overall severity of aphasia as measured by the Token Test had no influence. Surprisingly, the ratings of relatives were not sensitive to any of the aphasia variables, not even to reduction in expressive language. Thus, nonfluent aphasia seems to be better accepted by the relatives than by the patients themselves. This is seemingly at variance with a study by Zraick and Boone (1991), who reported for nonfluent aphasia a significantly higher number of negative attitudes of spouses towards the patient than for fluent aphasia.

Conclusions and further perspectives

These preliminary results are encouraging in that both the pictorial version for aphasic persons and the written proxy version given to their relatives appear to be useful and valid quality of life measures. The new pictorial version was shown to share strong psychometric properties with the more extensively studied written relatives' version. Some important features emerged in relation to factors that had clear impact on the quality of aphasic persons' lives.

First, the study makes it clear that both physical and psychosocial features contribute to perceived quality of life for this sample. A particular physical problem was the presence and extent of hemiparesis, as judged by both patients and their relatives. Interestingly non-aphasic family members perceived significantly more depression among their aphasic family members, an issue that needs further study. Second, age plays a significant role in all aspects of quality of life as measured here. Essentially older patients appeared to have more extensive physical problems as well as cognitive complaints, particularly as seen through relatives' eyes. Third, patients and relatives differed specifically on psychosocial, cognitive, and linguistic complaints. Relatives tended to indicate more such complaints than did their aphasic partners, but related them less frequently to degree and quality of the aphasic impairment. They seem to take a more functional perspective.

The sample under study here was highly selected and included only individuals who were largely independent for activities of daily living. In order to further study the clinical validity of the questionnaires, larger numbers of more impaired and less self-supportive aphasic individuals need to be studied.

REFERENCES

Aaronson, N. K. (1988). Quality of life: What is it? How should it be measured? *Oncology*, 2, 69–74.

Allison, P. J., Locker, D., & Feine, J. S. (1997). Quality of life: A dynamic construct. *Social Science in Medicine*, 45(2), 221–230.

Bergner, M., Bobitt, R. A., Carter, W. B., & Gilson, B. S. (1981). The Sickness Impact Profile: Development and final revision of a health status measure. *Medical Care*, 19, 787–805.

Borg, I. (1992). *Grundlagen und Ergebnisse der Facettentheorie*. Bern: Huber.

Carod-Artal, J., Egido, J. A., González, J. L., & de Seijas, V. (2000). Quality of life among stroke survivors evaluated 1 year after stroke. *Stroke*, 31, 2995–3000.

Damiano, A. M. (1996). *The Sickness Impact Profile. User's manual and interpretation guide*. Baltimore, MD: Johns Hopkins University.

de Haan, R., Aaronson, N., Limburg, M., Langton Hewer, R., & van Crevel, H. (1993). Measuring quality of life in stroke. *Stroke*, 24, 320–327.

de Haan, R. J., Limburg, M., van der Meulen, J. H. P., Jacobs, H. M., & Aaronson, N. K. (1995). Quality of life after stroke. Impact of stroke type and lesion location. *Stroke*, 26, 402–408.

Enderby, P., & Emerson, J. (1995). *Does speech and language therapy work? A review of the literature commissioned by the Department of Health*. London: Whurr.

Flanagan, J. C. (1982). Measurement of quality of life: Current state of the art. *Archives Psychological Medical Rehabilitation*, 63, 56–59.

Granger, C. V., Cotter, A. C., Hamilton, B. B., & Fiedler, R. C. (1993). Functional assessment scales: A study of persons after stroke. *Archives of Physical Medicine & Rehabilitation*, 74(2), 133–138.

Greener, J., Enderby, P., & Whurr, R. (2002). Speech and language therapy for aphasia following stroke (Cochrane Review). In *The Cochrane Library*, Issue 1. Oxford: Update Software.

Hoen, B., Thelander, M., & Worsley, J. (1997). Improvement in psychological well-being of people with aphasia and their families: Evaluation of a community-based programme. *Aphasiology*, 11(7), 681–691.

Huber, W., Poeck, K., Weniger, D., & Willmes, K. (1983). *Der Aachener Aphasie Test*. Göttingen: Hogrefe.

Huber, W., Poeck, K., & Willmes, K. (1985). The Aachen Aphasia Test. In F.C. Rose (Ed.), *Progress in aphasiology* (pp. 291–303). New York: Raven.

Huber, W., Springer, L., & Willmes, K. (1993). Approaches to aphasia therapy in Aachen. In A. Holland & M. Forbes (Eds.), *World perspectives on aphasia* (pp. 55–86). San Diego, CA: Singular.

Hütter, B. O. (2001). Sickness Impact Profile (SIP)—German version. In S. Salek (Ed.), *Compendium of quality of life instruments* . Chichester, UK: John Wiley & Sons.

Hütter, B. O., & Gilsbach, J. M. (1996). Das Aachener Lebensqualitätsinventar für Patienten mit Hirnschädigung: Entwicklung und methodische Gütekriterien. In H.J. Möller, R. Engel, & P. Hoff (Eds.), *Befunderhebung in der Psychiatrie: Lebensqualität, Negativsymptomatik und andere aktuelle Entwicklungen* (pp. 83–101). Berlin: Springer.

Hütter, B. O., & Würtemberger, G. (1997). Validity and reliability of the German version of the Sickness Impact Profile in patients with chronic obstructive pulmonary disease. *Psychology and Health*, 12, 149–159.

Katz, F. (1987). The science of quality of life. *Journal of Chronical Diseases*, 40(6), 459–463.

Kim, P., Warren, S., Madill, H., & Hadley, M. (1999). Quality of life of stroke survivors. *Quality of life research*, 8(4), 293–301.

King, R. B. (1996). Quality of life after stroke. *Stroke*, 27, 1467–1472.

Lingoes, J. C. (1979). Identifying region in the space for interpretation. In J. C. Lingoes, E. E. Roskam, & I. Borg (Eds.), *Geometric representation of relational data*. Ann Arbor, MI: Mathesis Press.

McNair, D. M., Lorr, M., & Droppelman, L. F. (1971). *Manual for the Profile of Mood States*. San Diego, CA: Educational and Industrial Testing Service.

Niemi, M. L., Laaksonen, R., Kotila, M., & Waltimo, O. (1988). Quality of life 4 years after stroke. *Stroke, 19*, 1101–1107.

Orley, J., & Kuyken, W. (1994). *Quality of life assessment: International perspectives*. Berlin: Springer.

Parker, C. J., Gladman, J. R., & Drummond, A. E. (1997). The role of leisure in stroke rehabilitation. *Disability and Rehabilitation, 19*(1), 1–5.

Pearson, V. A. H. (1995). Speech and language therapy: Is it effective? *Public Health, 109*, 143–153.

Poeck, K., Huber, W., & Willmes, K. (1989). Outcome of intensive speech therapy in aphasia. *Journal of Speech and Hearing Disorders, 54*, 471–479.

Robey, R. R. (1994). The efficacy of treatment for aphasic persons: A meta-analysis. *Brain and Language, 47*, 582–608.

Robey, R. R. (1998). A meta-analysis of clinical outcomes in the treatment of aphasia. *Journal of Speech, Language, and Hearing Research, 41*, 172–187.

Spitzer, W. O. (1987). State of science 1986. Quality of life and functional status as target variables for research. *Journal of Chronical Diseases, 40*(6), 465–471.

Stern, R. A., Arruda, J. E., Hooper, C. R., Wolfner, G. D., & Morey, C. E. (1997). Visual Analog Mood Scales to measure internal mood state in neurologically impaired patients: Description and initial validity evidence. *Aphasiology, 11*(1), 59–71.

Taylor Sarno, M. (1997). Quality of life in aphasia in the first post-stroke year. *Aphasiology, 11*(7), 665–679.

Visser, M. C. (1996). *Measurement of quality of life in patients with ischemic disease of the heart or brain*. Enschede: FEBRODRUK.

Zraick, R. I., & Boone, D. R. (1991). Spouse attitudes toward the person with aphasia. *Journal of Speech and Hearing Research, 34*, 123–128.

Reciprocal scaffolding: A context for communication treatment in aphasia

Jan R. Avent and Shannon Austermann

California State University, Hayward, USA

Background: The goal of social approaches to aphasia treatment is to improve life quality. This study explored the potential therapeutic value of increasing participation in life through natural language use with communicative partners during shared learning activities. Reciprocal Scaffolding Treatment (RST), based on an apprenticeship model of learning where novices are taught skills by a more skilled partner, was developed to provide an individual with aphasia an opportunity to use pre-stroke knowledge and vocabulary during teaching interactions.
Aims: The purposes of the study were to determine whether an individual with aphasia in the role as a teacher would improve language production and whether changes in quality of life were evident as a result of the experience.
Methods & Procedures: A descriptive case study approach was used to compare RST and peer discourse group treatment. The participant was a former physicist with moderate aphasia. He was placed in a preschool classroom to teach science to 4- and 5-year-old children. Correct information unit (CIU) analysis and type–token ratio (TTR) scores were used to compare language samples. Journal entries were used to document psychosocial and quality of life changes.
Outcomes & Results: Results indicated better verbal word retrieval skills within the classroom (RST) as compared to discourse group treatment. While involved in the teaching experience, the participant's lesson plans improved in detail and clarity. Journal entries showed improvements in quality of life.
Conclusions: These findings show how the re-application of prestroke vocational skills can enhance quality of life and improve language performance. While these results support a social approach to aphasia treatment, additional research is needed.

I believe that people identify things only in context.
                                    —John Steinbeck, *Travels with Charley* (1962)

Two words that seem to go together are "aphasia" and "change". Aphasia affects people in the midst of living their lives, and with little or no warning a person is thrust into a life that is permanently altered with immediate and long-lasting changes in employment, relationships, leisure activities, finances, and sense of self (Parr, Byng, Gilpin, & Ireland, 1997). This obviously causes a shift in psychosocial satisfaction (Byng, Pound, & Parr, 2000) and the quality of one's life.

Quality of life is a far-ranging concept including individual, social, and societal/community factors (Friedman, 1997). With respect to treatment, clinicians become advocates of quality of life by extending the scope of treatment beyond the clinic to include social and societal/community components. According to Friedrich in his book

Address correspondence to: Jan Avent, Communicative Sciences and Disorders, California State University, Hayward, Hayward, CA 94542, USA. Email: javent@csuhayward.edu

Successful Aging (2001), improvements in quality of life come about by intervening to prevent or reduce diseases, disorders, and disabilities; maintaining health and function; and enhancing societal roles, establishing interpersonal support, and reducing social isolation. These interventions for successful ageing are remarkably comparable to social approaches to aphasia treatment. Both address the needs to minimise disabilities, maintain function, and establish social connections.

The aim of social approaches to treatment is to enhance life quality. They are designed to improve communication (i.e., reduce disabilities and maintain function) and the psychosocial aspects (i.e., enhance societal roles, establish interpersonal support, and reduce social isolation) of aphasia (Avent, 1997; Lyon & Shadden, 2001; Simmons-Mackie, 2001). These approaches require that treatment be conducted in appropriate settings, involve real communication, recognise the reciprocal nature of communication between a sender and receiver, increase participation in life, and focus on both the interactional (social) and transactional (information exchange) characteristics of communication (Avent, 1997; Chapey, Duchan, Elman, Garcia, Kagan, & Lyon, 2000; Chapey et al., 2001; LaPointe, 1999; Lyon, 1999; Lyon & Shadden, 2001; Simmons-Mackie, 2001). Reciprocal Scaffolding Treatment (RST) was developed in our clinic at California State University, Hayward (CSUH) to explore the potential therapeutic value of increasing participation in life through natural language use with communicative partners during shared learning activities. The treatment focuses on an apprenticeship or reciprocal model of learning (Rogoff, 1990; Rogoff, Turkanis, & Bartlett, 2001), defined as learning that takes place in socially assembled situations where active novices (in this case children) learn skills and understanding through guided participation with more skilled partners (adults) (Rogoff, 1990). In RST, the more skilled partner is an adult with aphasia who is provided with an opportunity to use pre-stroke knowledge and vocabulary (Wepman, 1976) during routine teaching interactions with children (Bruner, 1983). The context for RST is designed to be mutually beneficial for the participants so that the aphasic individual teaches the novices a skill while the novices provide natural and complementary language models for the aphasic individual during genuine interactions, i.e., reciprocal support or scaffolding. To assess the effectiveness of this approach, an aphasic individual with a background in science was asked to develop and teach a curriculum to 4- to 5-year-old children. The purposes of the study were to determine (1) whether the aphasic participant's (AP) role as teacher affected his language production, and (2) whether changes in quality of life were evident as a result of the experience.

METHOD

This was a descriptive case study. Comparisons were made between data obtained from language samples collected during RST (science lesson with children) and group discourse treatment (peer participants). Additional data came from journals kept by one of the investigators (JA), the aphasic participant, and the spouse of the participant. AP was a 65-year-old man who was 21 months postonset of aphasia. His *Western Aphasia Battery* (Kertesz, 1982) AQ score was 75.7/100 and he typed with anomic aphasia. He received his BA and MSc degrees in physics, his PhD in nuclear engineering and his professional career included 28 years as a university professor. The treatment, comprising 10 science lessons with a group of young children, took place twice weekly for 6 weeks. In addition, AP received biweekly aphasia group treatment in the CSUH Aphasia Treatment Program. All RST (science lessons) and group discourse treatment sessions were held for 60 minutes to ensure a standard length of time (Malvern & Richards, 1997). AP prepared each science lesson independently. The science lessons occurred in a classroom of 25 children between the ages of 4 and 5 years at the Early Childhood Education Center (ECEC) at California State University, Hayward. Type–token ratios (TTR) (Retherford, 1993; Templin, 1957; Wachal & Spreen, 1973) and Correct Information Units (CIU) (Nicholas & Brookshire, 1993) were calculated for AP's language samples. AP and his spouse's descriptive journal entries were used to track potential psychosocial changes that may have occurred with treatment. There was no specific format for the journal entries.

RESULTS

Type–token ratio

AP's type–token ratios ranged from .15 to .41 during RST with an average of .23. His type–token ratios ranged from .14 to .21 during group discourse treatment with an average of .18. The TTR was higher during RST (science lessons with the children) than during the discourse group treatment interactions with peers. The results are reported in Table 1. These results show that AP used fewer total words (tokens) and fewer different words (types) during RST than during discourse treatment but lexical diversity was higher during RST. In addition, the range of lexical diversity was almost doubled during RST indicating a more powerful context for word retrieval. Overall, these findings suggest that the opportunity to use pre-stroke knowledge and vocabulary noticeably enhanced retrieval and use of a wider variety of words.

Correct information units

The average CIU score was higher during RST (science lessons) than the discourse interactions. In addition, the range of CIUs was different in the two contexts for treatment. There was almost no overlap in the two ranges with content consistently better during RST. The results are reported in Table 2. As with TTR measures, the number of total words and number of accurate content words (CIUs) were lower during RST compared to discourse treatment. Although fewer words were used during RST, the information was more accurate and suggests that this teaching experience was beneficial to improved communicative competence.

TABLE 1
TTRs calculated for RST and discourse group treatment

	Mean tokens	Mean types	TTR on means	Range of TTR
Reciprocal scaffolding treatment (science lesson with children)	419	89	0.23	.15–.41
Discourse group treatment (interactions with peers)	999	169	0.18	.14–.21

TABLE 2
CIUs calculated for RST and discourse group treatment

	Mean words	Mean CIUs	% of CIUs	Range of CIUs
Reciprocal scaffolding treatment (science lesson with children)	434	323	74	70–77%
Discourse group treatment (interactions with peers)	839	563	67	64–71%

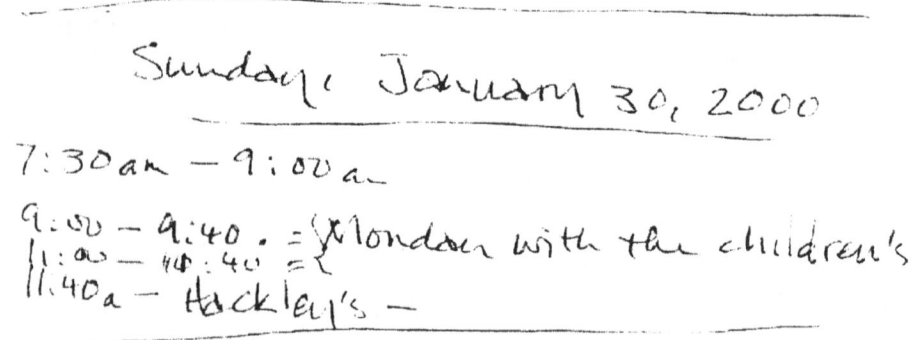

Figure 1.   AP's first journal entry pertaining to teaching.

Additional improvements

AP's journal entries for lesson planning became more thorough and complex over the course of treatment. The first journal entry pertaining to AP's teaching at the Early Childhood Education Center occurred on Sunday, January 30 with a brief notation of "9–9:40 a = Monday with the children's" (Figure 1). After his first week in the classroom, he began documenting his lesson plans in the schedule of his day. For the Saturday, February 5 entry, he listed the materials he would need for his science lesson, went to a movie, followed by additional notes about his science lesson (Figure 2). His lesson

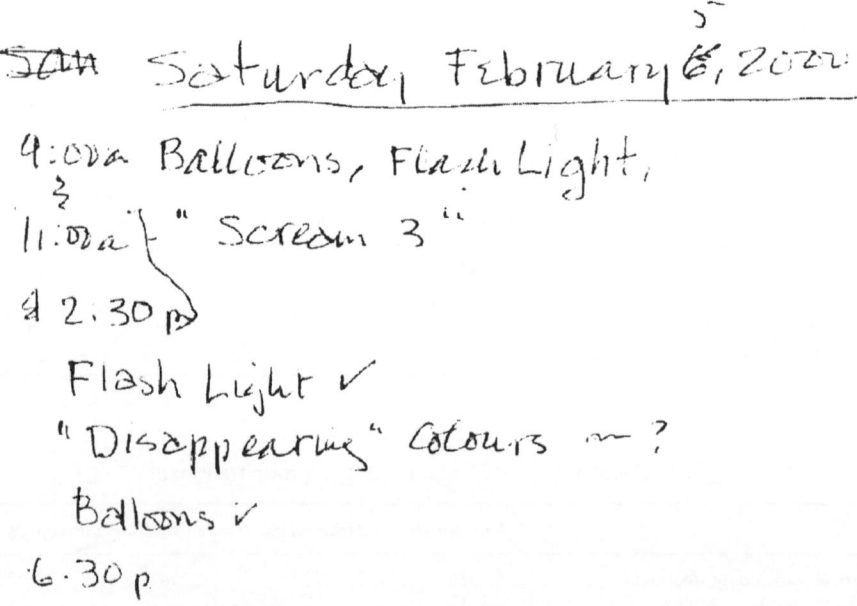

Figure 2.   AP's journal entry for Saturday, February 5.

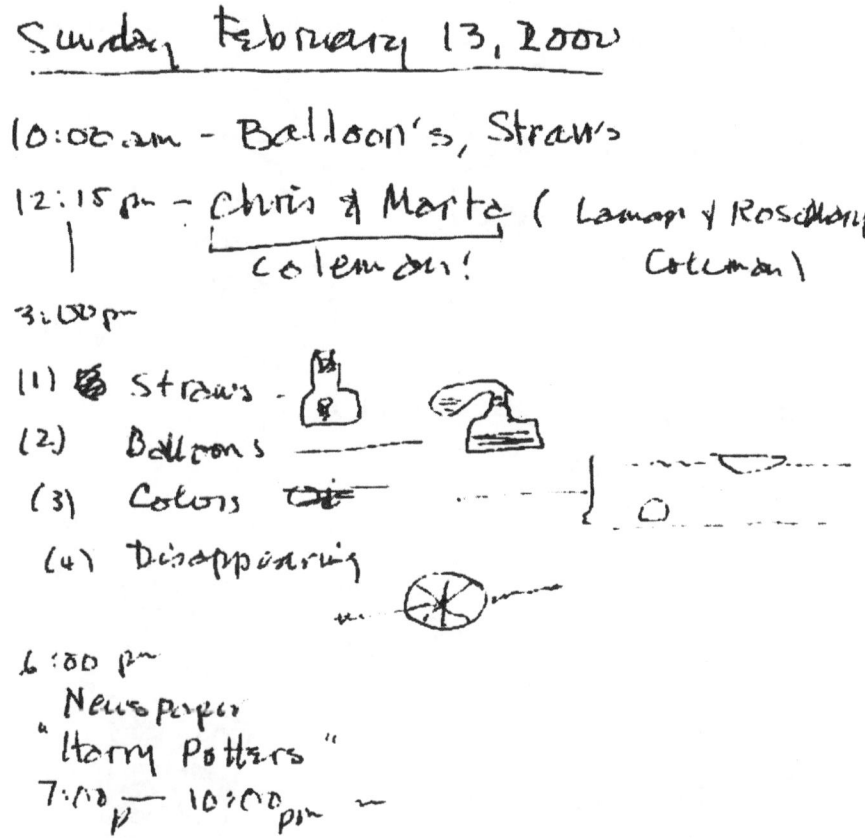

Figure 3. AP's journal entries begin to include simple conceptual drawings.

planning began to include simple conceptual drawings of experiments on February 13 (Figure 3), but the drawings became more elaborate with two- to four-part pictures for each experiment on February 16 (Figure 4). He further refined his lesson plan drawings by including improved written notations, although spelling and syntax errors were evident (e.g., "Friction causes vibrations on the *cub*" and "Weight of the offsets *very heaviest*") (Figure 5). These excerpts show how AP integrated his lesson planning in his daily activities at home and how he improved his conceptualisation and documentation of the science lessons over time.

Quality of life improvements

AP's spouse reported via her journal that the interactions with the children in the classroom coincided with AP's improved auditory comprehension of conversations in large groups, increased tolerance of noisy environments, and enhanced interactions with his grandchildren. Following completion of the study, AP was asked by the director of the ECEC to continue his teaching duties in the classroom. He accepted and continues to teach science at the Center.

Reliability.   The TTR and CIU data were independently scored by two of the researchers. Discrepancies were re-scored and 100% agreement was reached for both measures.

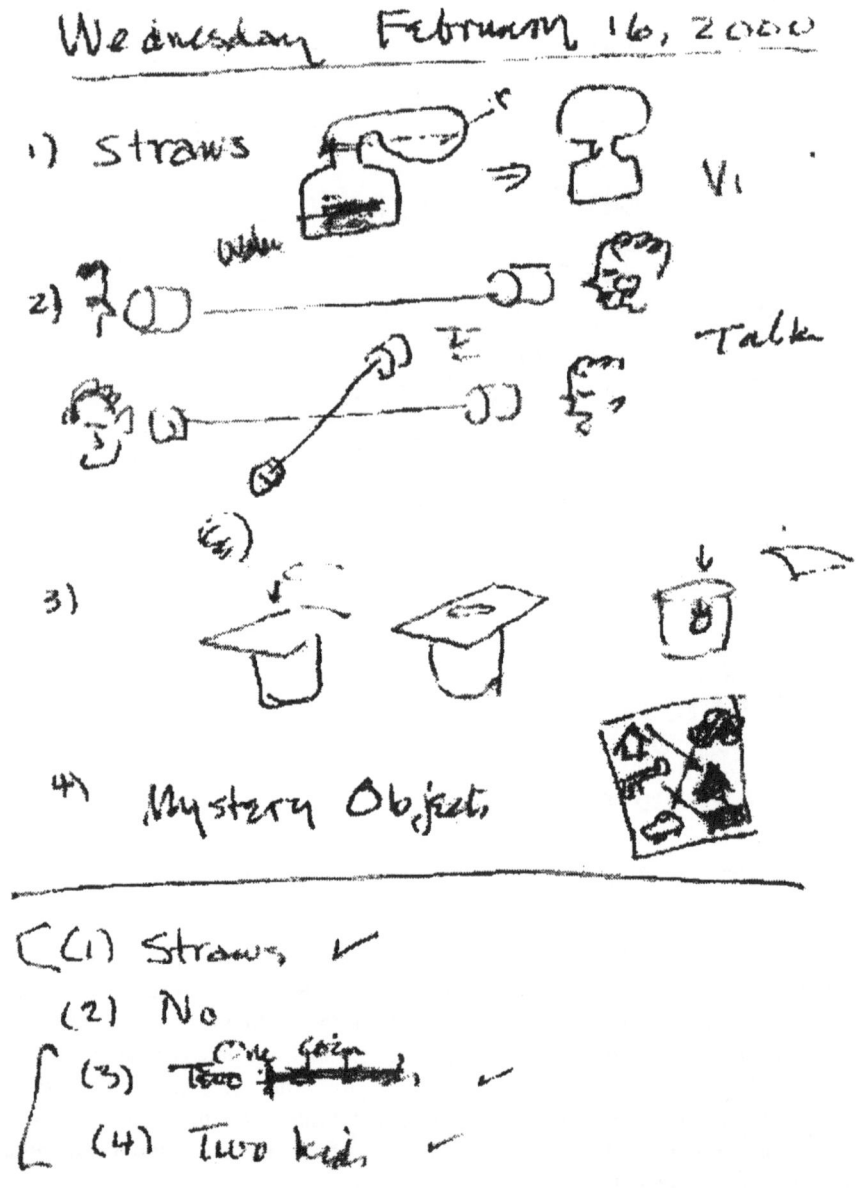

Figure 4.   More elaborate drawings.

DISCUSSION AND CONCLUSIONS

The purpose of this study was to explore whether RST would improve the language and life skills of an individual with aphasia. An aphasic individual (AP) with a background in science was asked to develop and teach a science curriculum to 4- and 5-year-old children. A case study approach was used to assess communication skills and changes in quality of life. Analysis of TTRs and CIUs revealed that the aphasic individual's vocabulary was more diverse and accurate during science lessons with children than during

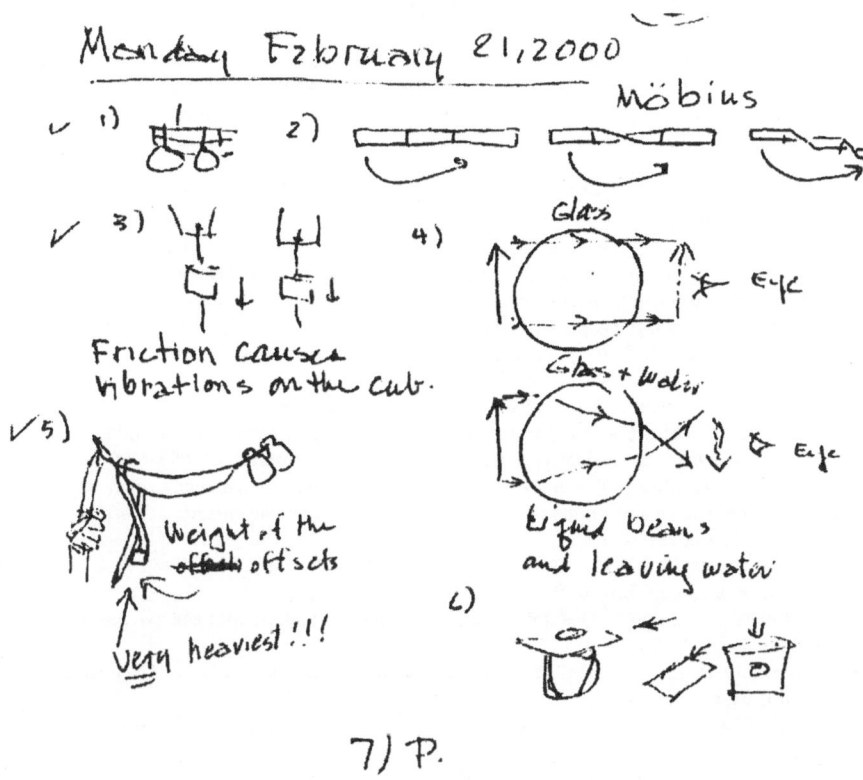

Figure 5.   Lesson plan drawings with written notations.

discourse sessions with peers. Journal entries related to the teaching experience showed improvements in written language skills and drawings as AP gained greater skill in his preparations for the classroom. Natural and complementary language interactions in the classroom corresponded to improved interactions with family and friends. These findings show how the re-application of strong pre-stroke skills through present reciprocal interactions such as teaching can accelerate psychosocial healing and language improvements and enhance self- and family-reported quality of life.

The value of a reciprocal scaffolding approach to social treatments is that it extends the therapeutic context of treatment to include mutually beneficial outcomes for all participants. As a result of RST, an aphasic individual gained greater access and use of familiar professional vocabulary, received authentic and complementary language models and feedback from his students in the classroom, was able to use his professional expertise, and improved his interactions with family and friends. He enjoyed the teaching and interactions with the children and found a new purpose in his life. The children acquired knowledge about science "from a real scientist" (their own description of AP).

Continued empirical validation is needed to define the scope and benefits of social approaches to treatment to overall quality of life. Results of this case study support social treatments of aphasia for enhancing quality of life and provide evidence of improved language and psychosocial skills as a result of Reciprocal Scaffolding Treatment.

REFERENCES

Avent, J. (1997). *Manual of Cooperative Group Treatment for Aphasia.* Boston, MA: Butterworth-Heinemann.

Bruner, J. (1983). *Child's talk: Learning to use language.* New York: W.W. Norton & Co.

Byng, S., Pound, C., & Parr, S. (2000). Living with aphasia: A framework for therapy interventions. In I. Papathanasious (Ed.), *Acquired neurogenic communication disorders: A clinical perspective.* London: Whurr Publishers.

Chapey, R., Duchan, J., Elman, R., Garcia, L., Kagan, A., & Lyon, J. (2000). Life participation approach to aphasia: A statement of values for the future. *Asha, 5,* 4–6.

Chapey, R., Duchan, J., Elman, R., Garcia, L., Kagan, A., Lyon, J., et al. (2001). Life participation approach to aphasia: A statement of values for the future. In R. Chapey (Ed.), *Language intervention strategies in aphasia and related neurogenic communication disorders.* Baltimore, MD: Lippincott Williams & Wilkins.

Friedman, M. I. (1997). *Improving the quality of life: A holistic scientific strategy.* Westport, CN: Praeger.

Friedrich, D. D. (2002). *Successful aging: Integrating contempory ideas, research findings, and intervention strategies.* Springfield, IL: Charles C. Thomas Publisher.

Kertesz, A. (1982). *Western Aphasia Battery.* New York: Grune & Stratton.

LaPointe, L. (1999). Quality of life with aphasia. *Seminars in Speech and Language, 20,* 5–18.

Lyon, J. (1999). A commentary on qualitative research in aphasia. *Aphasiology, 13,* 689–690.

Lyon, J., & Shadden, B. B. (2001). Treating life consequences of aphasia's chronicity. In R. Chapey (Ed.), *Language intervention strategies in aphasia and related neurogenic communication disorders.* Baltimore, MD: Lippincott Williams & Wilkins.

Malvern, D. D., & Richards, B. J. (1997). A new measure of lexical diversity. In A. Ryan & A. Wray (Eds.), *Evolving models of language.* Bristol, PA: Multilingual Matters Ltd.

Nicholas, L., & Brookshire, R. (1993). Quantifying connected speech of adults with aphasia. *Journal of Speech and Hearing Research, 36,* 338–350.

Parr, S., Byng, S., Gilpin, & Ireland, C. (1997). *Talking about aphasia: Living with loss of language after stroke.* London: Open University Press.

Retherford, K. S. (1993). *Guide to analysis of language transcripts* (2nd ed.). Eau Claire, WI: Thinking Publications.

Rogoff, B. (1990). *Apprenticeship in thinking: Cognitive development in social context.* New York: Oxford University Press.

Rogoff, B., Turkanis, C. G., & Bartlett, L. (2001). *Learning together: Children and adults in a school community.* New York: Oxford University Press.

Simmons-Mackie, N. (2001). Social approaches to aphasia intervention. In R. Chapey (Ed.), *Language intervention strategies in aphasia and related neurogenic communication disorders.* Baltimore, MD: Lippincott Williams & Wilkins.

Templin, M. C. *(1957). Certain language skills in children: Their development and interrelationships.* Minneapolis, MN: The University of Minnesota Press.

Wachal, R. S., & Spreen, O. (1973). Some measures of lexical diversity in aphasia and normal language performance. *Language and Speech, 16,* 169–181.

Wepman, J. (1976). Aphasia: Language without thought or thought without language. *Asha, 18,* 131–136.

APHASIOLOGY, 2003, *17* (4), 405–416

Viewing couples living with aphasia as adult learners: Implications for promoting quality of life

Riva Sorin-Peters

Ontario, Canada

Background: Current interventions for addressing the psychosocial consequences of aphasia have been based on professionally driven constructs as opposed to insider accounts of aphasia. An adult learning approach offers the possibility of developing a programme for individuals with aphasia and their families that involves a more holistic and person-centred approach. This approach offers insights about promoting the quality of life of couples living with aphasia.
Aims: The primary objective of this paper is to discuss the implications of adopting an adult learning approach in promoting the quality of life of couples living with chronic aphasia. This paper outlines current interventions for addressing the psychosocial consequences of aphasia. It describes an innovative approach of working with couples with aphasia that explicitly integrates adult education principles and strategies. The basic assumption of this approach is that learning begins with the learner, as opposed to the therapist or treatment plan.
Main Contribution: The main contribution of this paper is to outline an alternative approach to intervention that is based on an adult learning model. This approach suggests that improving quality of life for couples living with aphasia involves more than simply promoting increased participation in conversation. Placing the learner in the central role results in intervention goals that encompass emotional and marital issues, as well as communication.
Conclusions: The implications of the adult learning approach on promoting quality of life in the area of emotions, marital issues, and communication outcomes are discussed. Implications of this approach on the role of the speech-language pathologist are also examined.

The concept of "quality of life" as a scientific outcome measure represents the attempt to describe the overall results of communication assessment and intervention efforts in a way that is meaningful to both individuals with aphasia and speech-language pathologists. General definitions of quality of life vary in the literature and include dimensions related to physical, psychological, social, and spiritual factors (Calman, 1987; LaPointe, 1999; Spilker, 1990). However, there are concepts and ideas common to all definitions. The first is that quality of life is related to the individual's perception of performance. This represents a person-centred approach in which the individual serves as his/her own control, with comparisons made against expectation of function. The second is that the concept must be broad and cover all areas of life, including physical and occupational function, psychologic state, social interaction, and somatic sensation (Spilker, 1990). Third, all definitions emphasise the importance of personal growth and development to improve quality of life. Implicit in these concepts is the idea that quality of life will

Address correspondence to: Riva Sorin-Peters, 190 Winding Lane, Thornhill, Ontario, L4J 5J2, Canada. Email: rsorinpeters@rogers.com

© 2003 Taylor & Francis
http://www.tandf.co.uk/journals/pp/02687038.html   DOI:10.1080/02687030244000752

fluctuate over time as a result of changes in any or all of its component parts. It has also been considered important that such a definition be critically examined and tested.

Intrinsic to a definition of quality of life is a definition of health. The World Health Organisation defines health as a state of complete physical, mental, and social well-being and not merely the absence of disease or infirmity (Spilker, 1990). Translating this definition into more pragmatic terms for quality of life with brain damage that compromises communication is complex (King, 1996; LaPointe, 1999, 2000). Dimensions of quality of life are further complicated by the interactions imposed by individuality and culture. However, recent research has provided insight into some aspects of perceived quality of life after brain damage with communication loss. LeDorze and Brassard (1995) interviewed people with aphasia and their families. During and after discharge from traditional therapy, people with aphasia and their families reported decreased quality of life, social isolation, and inability to access former and new family and community activities. Several investigators have reported the impact of aphasia on psychosocial areas such as identity, self-esteem, relationships, and roles in the family (Byng, Pound, & Parr, 2000; Gainotti, 1997; Herrmann, 1997; Kagan, 1999). Parr (2001) interviewed 50 people living with long-term aphasia. Her "insider" perspective on aphasia suggests that its impacts are extensive and complex (Parr, 2001). Aphasia has an impact across the spectrum of social experience and the "psychosocial" problems associated with aphasia arise from a combination of internal and external factors. In addition, Parr (2001) found that the impacts of aphasia are both direct and indirect. Indirect consequences are evident in the difficulties people with aphasia have negotiating, legitimising, and managing the life changes that occur following stroke. The impacts of aphasia are interconnected; they are not separable, componential, or discrete. The impacts are also systemic; they are not experienced by the individual in isolation, but by numerous people in multiple contexts. Finally, the impacts of aphasia are dynamic, diversely experienced and continuous (Parr, 2001).

EXISTING PROGRAMMES FOR FAMILIES OF ADULTS WITH APHASIA

In response to the above, clinical approaches that integrate models of betterment of life quality in aphasia have been suggested (LaPointe, 1999; Parr, 2001). In this regard, family education (Helmick, Watamori, & Palmer, 1976; Williams, 1993), communication skills training (Alarcon, Hickey, Rogers, & Olswang, 1997; Olswang, Hickey, Alarcon, Rogers, Cadwell, & Schlegel, 1998; Simmons, Kearns, & Potechin, 1989; Wilkinson et al., 1998), and supportive counselling programmes (Holland, 2000; Johannsen-Horbach, Crone, & Wallesch, 1999; Nichols, Varchevker, & Pring, 1996; Wahrborg & Borenstein, 1989) have been reported as ways to complement traditional therapy.

Family education has been identified as important because family members tend to view the aphasic person's communication as less impaired than it most likely is (Helmick et al., 1976). This lack of understanding can lead to the establishment of unrealistic expectations for language performance and to the use of inappropriate amounts and types of language when interacting with the person with aphasia. However, although increased knowledge of aphasia may reduce the negative impact of stroke on caregivers (Williams, 1993), knowledge of aphasia alone is inadequate as a basis for coping with the associated problems (Linebaugh & Young-Charles, 1978).

Communication skills training programmes involve a shift from the role of the speech-language pathologist as a "fixer" of linguistic and/or cognitive aspects of communication deficits, to using speech-language pathology expertise to provide those who have aphasia with mutually satisfying conversation. In offering conversational opportunities, the role of the speech-language pathologist expands to include deliberate attempts to reduce frustration, with the aim of allowing participants to "forget" about the aphasia to the extent possible (Kagan, 1999). The implication of such approaches is that, by improving communication between aphasic adults and their family members, one may help improve social participation and mental well-being.

Lyon, Cariski, Keisler, Rosenbeck, and Levine (1997) have developed and implemented a Communication Partners programme that focuses on enhancing participation in life and communication in natural settings for adults with aphasia using triads of patient, caregiver, and a volunteer communication partner. Although scores on the Boston Diagnostic Aphasia Examination, Communication Abilities for Daily Living, or Affect Balance Scale did not yield statistically significant findings, patients and caregivers reported that the Communication Partners programme had improved their quality of life. Similarly, Kagan (1999) has developed and evaluated a Supported Conversation for Adults with Aphasia (SCA) programme for volunteers interacting with individuals with aphasia. Results have shown that training volunteers as conversation partners using a one-day workshop and 2 hours of hands-on experience is effective in improving the communication of volunteers and their partners with aphasia. However, this programme has not yet been applied to direct training of family members of adults with aphasia.

In this regard, Simmons et al. (1989) examined the effectiveness and generalisation of a spouse training programme for one couple. Results showed decreases in spouse interruptions and use of convergent questions, and suggest the usefulness of an individualised communication-oriented approach. Wilkinson et al. (1998) studied the effects of intervention that attempted to improve communication function between one couple by targeting patterns found in natural conversation between partners. Results showed a decrease in corrections, or "other-repairs", made by the spouse. Alarcon et al. (1997) have developed a Family Based Intervention for Chronic Aphasia (FICA) in which the person with aphasia and the spouse are more involved in assessment and evaluation. The focus of this intervention is on persistent communication problems between individuals with aphasia and their spouses, and the aim is to treat the disability in the context of typical interaction. Olswang et al. (1998) have found evidence of positive treatment effects of this intervention. These authors suggest that, although conversation involves only a dyad, the effects of aphasia involve the whole family system. Interventions therefore need to encompass the broader impact on the couple's relationship.

These studies suggest that communication training can help promote quality of life for couples by improving conversation. However, in the studies by Simmons et al. (1989), Wilkinson et al. (1998), and Olswang et al. (1998), participants began with a concrete experience which included a videotaped conversation, but the observations of these videotapes were largely influenced by the speech-language pathologist's perceptions of what constituted positive and negative communication behaviours. Training goals were determined by the clinicians, as opposed to being initiated by the couples. Clients were not actively involved in designing and evaluating the programme. Moreover, participants' emotions and marital issues were not explicitly addressed in the above studies.

Supportive counselling programmes have also been suggested in addressing the needs of individuals with aphasia and their families. Holland (2000) advocates the integration of counselling in individual work with adults with various neurogenic communication disorders at various states post-onset. She also discusses the need to provide counselling to families, both individually and in groups. Wahrborg and Borenstein (1989) have extended this counselling role to include family therapy with families with an aphasic member. Nichols et al. (1996) studied the effects of therapy given jointly by a family therapist and a speech-language pathologist. Johannsen-Horbach et al. (1999) attempted to address the needs of spouses of aphasic patients via both a nondirective counselling group and a group in which leaders used greater amounts of therapeutic interventions such as confrontation, interpretation, and clarification. Although positive changes in emotions and attitudes were documented in the above studies, these authors did not explicitly encourage participants to move from reflection towards the development of concepts about communication patterns that could then lead to applications in everyday life that would further improve quality of life.

Such programmes support the role of the speech-language pathologist in addressing the psychosocial sequelae of the aphasia. However, the alternative models and frameworks have been based on professionally driven constructs as opposed to insider accounts of aphasia. The literature represents the speech-language pathologist as the expert in a directive role. This emphasis on expertise rather than on a more holistic and person-centred approach to learning locates the source and power of change in the therapist, as opposed to in the person with aphasia and his or her family member. It is this very perspective that may be deflecting us from the real source of power to promote increased quality of life for these individuals. Further, the incorporation of a person-centred approach to communication and attitudes needs to be based on an explicit and well-organised theoretical framework.

AN ADULT LEARNING APPROACH

An adult learning approach offers the possibility of developing a programme for individuals with aphasia and their family members on a different basis that addresses the above issues. In this regard, a learner-centred training programme for spouses of adults with chronic aphasia has been developed and evaluated using a qualitative case study methodology (Sorin-Peters, 2002). The basic assumption in the development and implementation of this programme is that learning begins with the learner, as opposed to the therapist or treatment plan. Placing the learner in the central role involves more than a change in terminology and has significant ramifications for strategies to induce change.

The first phase of this learner-centred training programme for spouses of adults with chronic aphasia included the development of a training programme that integrated principles and strategies from speech-language pathology and adult education. One basic assumption of the adult learning approach is that the heart of education is learning, not teaching, so that the focus must shift from what the teacher does to what happens to the learner (Knowles, 1973). This is referred to by Hunt (1987) as "inside-out" learning, as opposed to "outside-in" learning. The programme's content was guided by adult learning principles and by insights gained from a needs assessment. The needs assessment confirmed that the explicit incorporation of adult education principles in the process of the programme was not only beneficial, but necessary in order to achieve success.

The second phase included the delivery and evaluation of the programme using a qualitative multiple case study methodology. This design resulted in a rich and holistic account of communication in couples with chronic aphasia and was useful in documenting change in complex communication behaviours after the training programme. Using videotaped conversations, the Couple Questionnaire (Olswang et al., 1998), and a semi-structured interview, this study examined changes in attitudes and communication behaviours in five couples immediately after training and at 2 months follow-up. All data were transcribed and analysed for patterns of change for each couple. An additional step in the data analysis was the development of a cross-case analysis.

Results indicated ways in which the adult learning principles were actualised across the five cases. Themes emerged related to the expression of emotions about aphasia. Themes related to marital issues also emerged and were intertwined with emotions and communication. Communication outcomes included positive changes in conversational repair, more balanced conversational control, the revealing of the competence of the partner with aphasia, and the emergence of different conversational genres that could be organised hierarchically. A paper, describing this study in detail, is currently under preparation (Sorin-Peters, 2003).

Unlike existing programmes, this programme includes all three components of education, communication skill training, and counselling. The data demonstrate that the integration of these three components was important in achieving the observed outcomes because each component was intimately related to the other. Moreover, this programme is unique in its explicit incorporation of adult learning principles as part of the process of the programme. In this approach, unlike in traditional medical model approaches, the client is seen as an experienced and competent adult learner and learning proceeds from his or her needs. Both members of the dyad are involved. Both are given more responsibility for goal selection and programme development. Clients become aware of their preferred learning styles and these preferences are taken into account throughout sessions.

The central role of spouses and partners in the learning process was actualised by using Kolb's experiential learning cycle model (Kolb, 1984) throughout sessions. Kolb's experiential learning cycle is displayed in Figure 1. Kolb's experiential learning cycle involves drawing on concrete experience, having participants engage in reflective observation, having participants engage in abstract conceptualisation, and encouraging participants to practise active experimentation in order to apply what they have learned. Although previous programmes have implicitly included various aspects of Kolb's learning model, none has explicitly incorporated all four activities in a systematic way. This programme began with spouses telling their "stories" about their experiences with

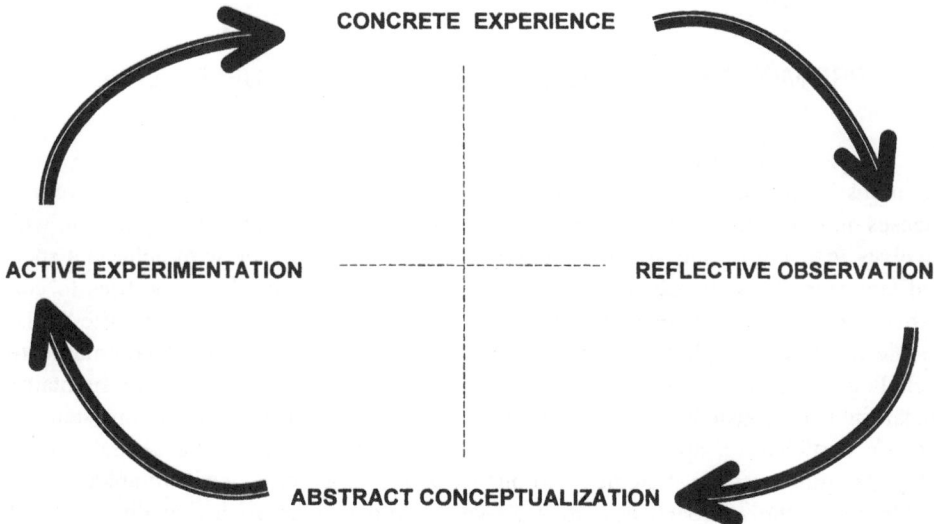

Figure 1.   Kolb's experiential learning cycle.

aphasia. Their previous knowledge about aphasia as well as their use of communication techniques that had been working well were affirmed. The use of reflective learning questions helped spouses to systematically review their experiences with aphasia in order to understand how it was impacting communication with their partners. Their reflections served as the basis for them to collaborate in setting goals and designing the programme agenda. They were assisted in developing new or revised concepts about aphasia and ways to facilitate communication with their partners. Spouses were assisted in applying this information to improve the quality of communication with their partners. This involved identifying and addressing their learning styles and diversity of needs. It also involved making adjustments based on their rhythms of learning and building on the unexpected. Self-evaluations helped empower couples to monitor their performance and continue to learn after the programme had ended. By thus incorporating all four processes of experience, reflection, conceptualisation, and application into the programme, more fully integrated and transformational learning was able to occur. This is consistent with the intent of Kolb's learning cycle (Kolb, 1984), which is to promote a process of learning through critical self-reflection on experience. It differs from the traditional approach of having the speech-language pathologist predetermine appropriate techniques and then teach these to spouses.

The incorporation of adult education principles adds a new dimension to intervention. The elements of sharing their experience, reflecting on their experience, and conceptualising and applying what had been learned resulted in the surfacing of emotions and marital issues that impacted on communication. Adult education principles appeared to help bridge these three components of intervention naturally, in a way that could not have been attained without their use. Placing the learner in the central role also prompted the development of a broad and holistic scope of intervention. More than one aspect of spouses' and partners' learning capacities were tapped throughout the training. These included emotional, relational, physical, intellectual, and intuitive capabilities. The holistic learning approach in this programme involved looking at communication behaviours in the context of the couple and family system, and treating the structure as a whole.

This approach appeared to offer insights about promoting the quality of life of couples living with aphasia.

PROMOTING THE QUALITY OF LIFE OF COUPLES LIVING WITH APHASIA

The life participation approach to aphasia (Chapey, Duchan, Garcia, Kagan, Lyon, & Simmons-Mackie, 2000) refers to a general philosophy and model of service delivery that focuses on re-engagement in life. It represents a shift from the remedial approach, which involves focusing on the impairment and disability of the person with aphasia's speech and language skills. It goes beyond compensatory instruction where one tries to counterbalance or substitute one skill for another. It involves a focus on the real-life goals of people affected by aphasia. It recommends that the dual function of communication including transmitting and receiving messages, as well as establishing and maintaining social links, be considered. In order to promote communication changes consistent with the life participation approach, we need to place the learner in the central role and integrate adult learning strategies into our work with couples living with aphasia.

Moreover, the approach described above showed that improving quality of life for couples living with aphasia involves more than simply promoting increased participation in conversation. Placing the learner in the central role resulted in intervention goals that encompassed emotional and marital issues, as well as communication.

EXPRESSING EMOTIONS

The adult learning approach begins with people sharing their experiences of living with a partner with aphasia and reflecting on this experience. This facilitates the expression of feelings about the aphasia. These emotions may include anger, sadness and grief, and acceptance.

The expression of anger

Several couples initially expressed feelings of anger and resentment related to the consequences of the aphasia. For example, one partner with aphasia overtly expressed intense anger and shouted at his partner during initial sessions. These emotions were acknowledged and this partner was made aware of how his anger was negatively impacting on his relationship with his wife. He was encouraged to reflect on these feelings and to express his feelings to his wife in a respectful and loving way.

Being aware of the possibility that couples may have angry feelings can prepare speech-language pathologists for the outpouring of anger and resentment that may accompany the exploration of new communication techniques. It is important to see the expression of such emotions as a natural accompaniment to change, and to allow time for their expression. If feelings of anger in learners are repressed, they may fester until they represent a much larger block to learning (Brookfield, 1990). Recognising that anger can block learning suggests the importance of emotional support throughout a communication training programme.

The expression of sadness and grief

In addition to anger, all spouses expressed sadness about the consequences of the aphasia and alluded to feeling grief because of losses. For example, one spouse commented that it was harder to live with a partner with aphasia than to cope with the death of one's partner. While the partners were still physically present, their inability to communicate with their spouses in the same way as before the stroke had produced a gap in the relationship. This is consistent with the concept of "ambiguous loss" (Boss, 1991), which includes the psychological loss of a family member even though they are physically present. For these spouses, dealing with the consequences of the stroke and resulting aphasia was not a transitory process, but a permanent state and lifestyle. It would be helpful for clinicians to acknowledge this ambiguity to spouses and families of adults with aphasia. Moreover, it is important to help couples move beyond these feelings by explaining and demonstrating to spouses how the partner with aphasia can still be included in conversations, thus promoting his or her inclusion in the family system. This, in turn, may help spouses to set new boundaries, reassign roles, and take charge in new ways, thereby promoting resiliency and the reconstruction of family life.

Increased acceptance of the aphasia after training

Luterman (1995) describes four phases in the acceptance process of chronic illness. These include denial, resistance, affirmation, and integration. By agreeing to participate in the training, couples implicitly acknowledged that their partners had aphasia and that they were willing to accept help; they had thereby reached the affirmation phase. Luterman points out that this stage is characterised by a great deal of pain, as there is an acceptance of the notion that things will never be as they previously had been. In turn, this implies that, even when couples are willing to accept help, it is important to support them emotionally. Moreover, there is a need for intervention in the ''affirmation'' phase as it is possible to help couples move beyond this phase via a learner-centred programme. With training, couples developed new or modified ways of communicating. They were then able to move towards the ''integration'' stage where they could deal with the aphasia and participate in other activities. This involved the need for them to come to a deeper acceptance of the aphasia, learning to live with it by integrating the new communication strategies into their conversations, and then moving on to focus on other matters.

To promote quality of life for couples living with aphasia, we need to address emotional issues that may block learning. We need to allow couples to express feelings of anger and grief. We can also systematically help them move towards an increased acceptance of the consequences of aphasia.

MARITAL ISSUES

The adoption of an adult learning approach requires the application of a systems approach whereby each couple is viewed as more than the sum of its two parts. The whole consists of all the parts *plus* the way the parts operate in relation to one another. The couple is seen as an interacting network in which each member influences the nature of the entire system and in turn is influenced by it. One implication of such an approach is that when one part of a family system is ''damaged'' in some way, then every part is affected. This means that when one member of a family has aphasia, all members of the family are influenced by it.

The use of the adult learning strategies consistent with this systems approach resulted in the surfacing of marital issues. Such issues were intertwined with feelings about aphasia and with communication. These issues were dealt with because they appeared to have an impact on communication issues, and progress in communication would be limited if they were not addressed. It seemed as though the communication issues were superficial and that the emotions and marital issues were deeply rooted but intimately connected to the communication problems. Once these deeper issues were addressed in some way, the communication training flowed smoothly. Examples of intervention goals involving marital issues include couples finding new ways of spending time with each other, couples setting aside time for conversation, couples wanting to have their partners express appreciation or gratitude to each other, and couples needing to have their partners show affection towards them.

To promote quality of life for couples with aphasia, we need to address marital issues that are intertwined with communication. Research in marital therapy has outlined five types of relationship maintenance behaviours that function to preserve ongoing relationships (Canary & Stafford, 1992). These include positivity, openness, assurances, network, and the sharing of tasks (Canary & Stafford, 1992). The use of these maintenance behaviours is associated with higher perceptions of satisfaction, commitment, and liking which are all key indicators of relationship quality (Canary & Stafford, 1994). The present approach demonstrated that learner-centred training can promote the development of relationship maintenance behaviours for couples who are willing to commit to interventions such as this one.

COMMUNICATION OUTCOMES

Viewing couples as adult learners warrants the modification of supported conversation programmes, such as that developed by Kagan (1999) for volunteers. In contrast to Kagan's group format for training volunteers (1999), spouses need to be seen either individually or with their partners in order to address couples' specific needs. Adult learning principles should be explicitly incorporated. In the current example, it involved using Kolb's experiential learning cycle throughout sessions. Emotional and marital issues may surface and need to be addressed. Follow-up is beneficial to monitor progress and to maintain or further improve the quality of communication between couples.

The approach described here demonstrated that the wider scope of a learner-centred programme can promote a wider scope of communication changes for couples living with aphasia. These include, first, improvements in interaction and the transaction of information in conversation as well as increases in aphasic partners' participation in conversation. Second, the cognitive competence of the partner with aphasia was revealed through the skill of the trained spouse in conversation. Third, communication changes using an adult learning approach included more balanced topic, turn, and response control in conversation. Finally, a hierarchy of different conversation genres emerged, moving from conversation that was focused on the performance of the partner to conversation with more topic elaboration. All spouses initially "tested" their partners. After intervention, communication developed to include reminiscences and discussions. Such reminiscences included both members of the couple sharing a memory of an experience. These reminiscences changed the whole tenor of the conversation. This suggests that reminiscence, when used with appropriate conversation strategies, can be a powerful conversation tool for couples. A higher level of conversation included discussions of ideas and opinions or new information, such as gardening issues, issues related to children, and issues about relatives.

By improving the quality of communication between couples, the quality of the relationship also seems to improve, thereby promoting improved quality of life. For example, one spouse said afterwards that not only was her partner communicating better, but also there was a smaller gap between them and between her partner and their children. Her improved ability to communicate with him also resulted in him helping more with errands and domestic chores, thereby reducing her domestic responsibilities. Another spouse said that, as a result of improved communication with his partner, he was more like the way he used to be before the stroke; he was demonstrating his sense of humour and beginning to joke more with his wife.

IMPLICATIONS REGARDING THE ROLE OF THE SPEECH-LANGUAGE PATHOLOGIST

The adoption of an adult learning approach expands the speech-language pathologist's role to one of helping spouses and couples make their own meaning of the consequences of the aphasia, by moving them through the four phases of the experiential learning cycle (Figure 1). This can foster a growing acceptance and ability to develop creative solutions that can be applied at home and, eventually, can be developed and applied without the speech-language pathologist's direct involvement. These changes can promote increased quality of life for couples living with aphasia.

The adult learning approach of aphasia thus extends the existing psychosocial model by focusing on the importance of communication for the expression of emotions and the maintenance and development of marital relations. This philosophy of practice represents a more comprehensive approach in our work and explicitly acknowledges the influence of communication on the expression of emotions and marital issues. When any aspect of communication, emotion, or marital relations is addressed, it impacts on the other in a holistic way. This results in outcomes that include more than increased participation in communication—the outcome is characterised by a more global feeling of overall well-being. Thus, rather than aiming intervention at the impairment, activity, or even participation levels, the adult learning model approach promotes a broader and deeper approach to the couple system and results in more comprehensive changes of wellness.

We need to get to know the learner's world; his/her feelings, experiences, and perceptions of his/her experiences. When we begin our interventions by listening to individuals' stories and experiences, and acknowledging their feelings and challenges, we can help individuals to reflect on these experiences so that they can become critically aware of their old assumptions and perspectives. We can acknowledge attitudes and behaviours that are serving them well and help them see options for dealing with the constraints imposed by the aphasia which may have previously been perceived as beyond their control. By adding knowledge, skills, or increasing competencies to these new perspectives, we increase the possibility for a plan of action that results in more holistic and lasting changes. We thereby encourage individuals with aphasia and their spouses to move forward to new perspectives and behaviours, while building competence and confidence in these new roles and relationships.

We suggest here the expansion of the speech-language pathologist's role from a conversation partner or facilitator in enhancing access to life participation via conversation, to that of a more active participant in the change process. The use of the adult learning approach requires the speech-language pathologist to be open to a broad range of client behaviour, such as emotions and marital issues. It requires that one be nonjudgemental and to maintain one's regard for the couple despite their particular choices and characteristics.

Such increased personal involvement will permit the speech-language pathologist's own feelings and issues to arise. He/she will become more involved subjectively and will need to use feelings and intuition as guides to the change process. In fact, speech-language pathologists themselves will be involved in their own experiential learning cycles when adopting this approach. This implies that in order to help spouses and adults with aphasia move through the experiential learning cycle, we need to become comfortable and confident in our own movement through this cycle. Similarly, just as the adult learning approach permits couples to become aware of and use the learning potential of their emotional, relational, physical, and intuitive capabilities in their own learning, speech-language pathologists can become more aware of these learning capabilities within themselves and thereby tap into these capabilities to promote more comprehensive and meaningful changes in spouses and adults with aphasia.

CONCLUSION

Parr's (2001) qualitative work on the psychosocial aspects of aphasia suggests the advantage of an "insider", versus an "outsider", perspective. An "insider" approach focuses on the perspectives of people with aphasia and addresses the "illness", not the "disease" of aphasia. The adult learning approach to intervention described in this paper represents an alternative model to intervention that is based on insider accounts of aphasia. The learner-centred approach is not prescriptive, but rather represents an alternate process of intervention. The central role of the learner results in goals, activities, and outcomes that are developed by the learner. This results in changes in emotions and marital issues, as well as communication, that are specific and meaningful to the individual learners. The competence of the individual with aphasia and his/her family to learn is explicitly acknowledged in this approach, thereby enhancing self-esteem and the ability to continue learning after intervention.

The adult learning model suggests a relationship in which the speech-language pathologist and couple are active collaborators in the learning process. For speech-language pathologists to utilise this approach, we may need to widen our technical expertise and learn more about adult education principles and their application to our work. We may also need to learn more about family systems and marital interactions and ways of dealing with interactions in families in intervention programmes. We also need to trust and develop our intuitive capabilities and "inner wisdom". In order to do this, clinicians may need to rely on the "art" of their work and trust their interpretations. By widening our technical expertise and also trusting and developing our own inner wisdom, we may better share some of the "walk" with our clients and facilitate more meaningful changes, thereby promoting improved quality of life.

REFERENCES

Alarcon, N., Hickey, E., Rogers, M., & Olswang, L. (1997). *Family based Intervention for Chronic Aphasia (FICA): An alternate service delivery model.* Presentation given at Non-Traditional Approaches to Aphasia Conference, Yountville, California.

Boss, P. (1991). Ambiguous loss. In F. Walsh, & M. McGoldrick (Eds.), *Living beyond loss: Death in the family.* New York: W.W. Norton & Company.

Brookfield, S. (1990). *The skillful teacher.* San Fransisco: Josey-Bass.

Byng, S., Pound, C., & Parr, S. (2000). Living with aphasia: A framework for interventions. In I. Papathanasiou (Ed.), *Acquired neurogenic communication disorders: A clinical perspective.* London: Whurr.

Calman, K. C. (1987). Definitions and dimensions of quality of life. In N. K. Aaronson & J. H. Beckmann (Eds.), *The quality of life of cancer patients.* New York: Raven Press.

Canary, D. J., & Stafford, L. (1992). Relational maintenance strategies and equity in marriage. *Communication Monographs, 59,* 243–1267.

Canary, D. J., & Stafford, L. (1994). Maintaining relationships through strategic and routine interaction. In D. J. Canary, & L. Stafford (Eds.), *Communication and relational maintenance.* San Diego: Academic Press, Inc.

Chapey, R., Duchan, J. F., Garcia, L. J., Kagan, A., Lyon, J., & Simmons-Mackie, N. (2000). Life participation approach to aphasia: A statement of values for the future. *The ASHA Leader, 5*(3), 4–6.

Gainotti, G. (1997). Emotional, psychological, and psychosocial consequences of aphasic patients: An introduction. *Aphasiology, 11*(7), 635–650.

Helmick, J. W., Watamori, T. S., & Palmer, J. M. (1976). Spouses' understanding of the communication disabilities of aphasic patients. *Journal of Speech and Hearing Disorders, 41,* 238–243.

Hermann, M. (1997). Studying psychosocial problems in aphasia: Some conceptual and methodological considerations. *Aphasiology, 11,* 717–725.

Holland, A. (2000). *Counselling individuals with neurogenic communication disorders.* McGeachy Memorial Lecture. Department of Speech-Language Pathology: University of Toronto, Canada.

Hunt, D. E. (1987). *Beginning with ourselves: In practice, theory, and human affairs.* Toronto: OISE Press.

Johannsen-Horbach, H., Crone, M., & Wallesch, C. W. (1999). Group therapy for spouses of aphasic patients. *Seminars in Speech and Language, 20*(1), 73–83.

Kagan, A. (1999). *'Supported conversation for adults with aphasia': Methods and evaluation.* Doctoral thesis, Institute of Medical Science, University of Toronto.

King, R. B. (1996). Quality of life after stroke. *Stroke, 27*(9), 1467–1472.

Knowles, M. S. (1973). *The adult learner: A neglected species.* Houston, TX: Gulf Publishing Company.

Kolb, D. A. (1984). *Experiential learning: Experience as the source of learning and development.* Englewood Cliffs, NJ: Prentice Hall, Inc.

LaPointe, L. L. (1999). Quality of life with aphasia. *Seminars in Speech and Language, 20*(1), 5–17.

LaPointe, L. L. (2000). Quality of life with brain damage. *Brain and Language, 71,* 135–137.

LeDorze, G., & Brassard, C. (1995). A description of the consequences of aphasia on aphasic persons and their relatives based on the WHO model of chronic disease. *Aphasiology, 9*(3), 239–255.

Linebaugh, C. W., & Young-Charles, H. Y. (1978). The counselling needs of families of aphasic patients. In R. K. Brookshire (Ed.), *Clinical Aphasiology Conference Proceedings*. Minneapolis, Minnesota: BRK Publishers.

Luterman, D. (1995). *In the shadows: Living and coping with a loved one's chronic illness*. Bedford, MA: Jade Press.

Lyon, J. G., Cariski, D., Keisler, L., Rosenbeck, J., & Levine, R. (1997). Communication partners: Enhancing participation in life and communication for adults with aphasia in natural settings. *Aphasiology, 11*(7), 693–708.

Nichols, F., Varchevker, A., & Pring, T. (1996). Working with people with aphasia and their families: An exploration of the use of family therapy techniques. *Aphasiology, 10*(8), 767–781.

Olswang, L., Hickey, E., Alarcon, N., Rogers, M., Cadwell, C., & Schlegel, E. (1998). *Treating the disability: measurement issues in efficacy research*. Unpublished research, University of Washington, USA.

Parr, S. (2001). Psychosocial aspects of aphasia: Whose perspectives? *Folia Phoniatrica et Logopaedica, 53*, 266–288.

Simmons, N. N., Kearns, K. P., & Potechin, G. (1989). Treatment of aphasia through family member training. In T. Prescott (Ed.), *Clinical Aphasiology Conference Proceedings*. San Diego: College-Hill Press.

Sorin-Peters, R. (2002). *The development and evaluation of a learner-centred training program for spouses of adults with chronic aphasia*. Doctoral thesis, University of Toronto, Canada.

Sorin-Peters, R. (2003). The evaluation of a learner-centred training program for spouses of adults with chronic aphasia. Manuscript in preparation.

Spilker, B. (1990). *Quality of life assessments in clinical trials*. New York: Raven Press.

Wahrborg, P., & Borenstein, P. (1989). Family therapy with an aphasic member. *Aphasiology, 3*(1), 93–98.

Wilkinson, R., Bryan, K., Lock, S., Bayley, K., Maxim, J., Bruce, C., Edmundson, A., & Moir, D. (1998). Therapy using conversation analysis: Helping couples adapt to aphasia in conversation. *International Journal of Language and Communication Disorders, 33* (Suppl), 144–149.

Williams, S. E. (1993). The impact of aphasia on marital satisfaction. *Archives of Physical Medicine and Rehabilitation, 74*, 3611–367.

APHASIOLOGY

APHASIOLOGY is covered by the following abstracting and indexing services: *BLLDB (Bibliography of Linguistic Literature), Current Contents: Clinical Medicine, EMBASE/Excerpta Medica, Linguistic Abstracts, Linguistic and Language Behavior Abstracts, Medical Documentation Service, Neuroscience Citation Index, PsychInfo, Research Alert, SciSearch, UnCover.*

Submitting a paper to   APHASIOLOGY

Aphasiology is concerned with all aspects of language impairment and related disorders resulting from brain damage. Submissions are encouraged on theoretical, empirical and clinical topics from any disciplinary perspective, and submissions which involve cross disciplinary study are particularly welcome. *Aphasiology* will publish experimental and clinical research papers, reviews, theoretical notes, comments and critiques. Research reports can be group studies, single-case studies or surveys, on psychological, linguistic, medical and social aspects of aphasia. Submissions and ideas for the Review Articles and the Forum are welcome and interdisciplinary peer commentary is encouraged.

Structured Abstracts.

Authors submitting papers should note that from Volume 16 Issue 1 (2002), the journal is introducing Structured Abstracts. There is good evidence that Structured Abstracts are clearer for readers and facilitate better appropriate indexing and citation of papers.

The essential features of the Structured Abstract are given below. Note in particular that any clinical implications should be clearly stated.

Abstract (Between 150-400 words)

Background: Describe the background to the study;

Aims: State the aims and objectives of the study including any clear research questions or hypotheses.

Methods & Procedures: To include outline of the methodology and design of experiments; materials employed and subject/participant numbers with basic relevant demographic information; the nature of the analyses performed.

Outcomes & Results: Outline the important and relevant results of the analyses.

Conclusions: State the basic conclusions and implications of the study. State, clearly and usefully, if there are implications for management, treatment or service delivery.

Review Abstract

Background: Outline the background to the review.

Aims: State the primary objective of the paper; the reasons behind your critical review and analyses of the literature; your approach and methods if relevant.

Main Contribution: The main outcomes of the paper and results of analyses; and any implications for future research and for management, treatment or service delivery.

Conclusions: State your main conclusions.

Papers for consideration should be sent to an Editor. Please send an original and three photocopies. Do not send original MRI scans until accepted for publication.

Papers are accepted for consideration on condition that you will accept and warrant the following conditions:

1. You will transfer copyright to Psychology Press Ltd, should the work be accepted for publication.
2. The work is your original work, and cannot be construed as plagiarising any other published work.
3. You own the copyright in the work.
4. You are empowered by your fellow author(s) to make a submission to this journal, and to make any agreement relating to the work.
5. Your work has not previously been published in the English language.
6. Your work is not under consideration for publication elsewhere, in any form.
7. You have secured the necessary permission in writing from the appropriate authorities for the reproduction in your work of any text, illustration, or other material which is reproduced or derived from a copyrighted source.
8. You have agreed with your fellow author(s) the order of names for publication of the work.
9. You warrant that the work does not include content that is abusive, defamatory, libellous, obscene, fraudulent, or in violation of applicable laws.

If it is found acceptable for publication, you shall retain the right to use the substance of the above work in future works, on condition that you acknowledge its prior publication in the journal, and to the publishers Psychology Press Ltd.

Fifty complimentary offprints of the article and a complimentary copy of the issue in which your article appears will be sent to the principal or sole author of articles; book reviewers will be sent three copies of the issue free of charge. Larger quantities of offprints may be ordered at a special discount price. An order form will accompany the proof.

Submissions and books for, or offers to, review should be sent to an Editor, address on inside front cover.

Style Guides

Please refer to the following website for the journal style guide, and for more information on our other journals and books: http://www.psypress.co.uk